Tom,

This is a biography of your great-great grandfather. It caused some conmon in the family as it recorded an event involving your great-grandfather. Read it find out about it.

Love Dad.

EPONYMISTS IN MEDICINE

John Langdon Down
1828–1896

A Caring Pioneer

O Conor Ward

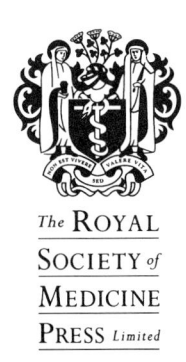

The ROYAL
SOCIETY of
MEDICINE
PRESS Limited

©1998 Royal Society of Medicine Press Ltd
1 Wimpole Street, London W1M 8AE, UK
16 East 69th Street, New York, NY 10021, USA

Apart from any fair dealing for the purpose of research or private study, criticism or review, as permitted under the UK Copyright, Designs and Patents Act, 1988, no part of this publication may be reproduced, stored, or transmitted, in any form or by any means, without the prior permission in writing of the publishers or in the case of reprographic reproduction in accordance with the terms of licenses issued by the Copyright Licensing Agency in the UK, or in accordance with the terms of licenses issued by the appropriate Reproduction Rights Organization outside the UK. Enquiries concerning reproduction outside the terms stated here should be sent to the publishers at the UK address printed on this page.

British Library Cataloguing in Publication Data
A catalogue record for this book is available from the British Library

ISBN 1-85315-374-5

Phototypeset by Dobbie Typesetting Limited, Tavistock, Devon

Printed in Great Britain by Henry Ling Ltd, the Dorset Press, Dorchester, Dorset

To Pauline, constant companion for 50 years.

... the perfect wife. She is far beyond the price of rubies.
(Old Testament. Pr.31;10)

Contents

List of Illustrations		vii
Table of Events		xi
Acknowledgements		xiii
Foreword		xv
Introduction		xvii
Chapter 1	Early Life	1
Chapter 2	The Pharmaceutical Chemist	7
Chapter 3	Return to Torpoint	15
Chapter 4	To Medical School	19
Chapter 5	The Royal Earlswood Asylum for Idiots	29
Chapter 6	Life in Earlswood and the Reforms	41
Chapter 7	Family Affairs	53
Chapter 8	Dealing and Doctoring in Earlswood	61
Chapter 9	Normansfield	77
Chapter 10	Development of Normansfield	95
Chapter 11	The Mistress of Normansfield	107
Chapter 12	Sundays, Weekdays and Entertainment	115
Chapter 13	A Death in the Family	123
Chapter 14	Down's Syndrome	129
Chapter 15	Reginald and Percival Langdon Down	139
Chapter 16	Down's Syndrome Patients in Normansfield	149
Chapter 17	The Lettsomian Lectures and Other Papers	157
Chapter 18	Down's Influences and Beliefs	175
Chapter 19	The Langdon Down Photographs	187
Chapter 20	The End of a Partnership	195
Chapter 21	Fame after Death	199
Appendix 1	Indenture of John Langdon Down to his father as an apothecary, 1849	203
Appendix 2	A History of the Normansfield Theatre, by John Earl	205
Index		209

List of Illustrations

Plan of Torpoint houses. All were built to the same design in narrow streets. (Courtesy of Sir Richard Carew Pole) — 3

The Pharmaceutical Society in 1845. (Courtesy of Royal Pharmaceutical Society) — 9

Advertising flyer for Richard Down's diarrhoea mixture — 12

Dr WJ Little, a senior physician at the London Hospital, presented Langdon Down with an inscribed copy of his famous text book. The inscription reads: 'JH Langdon Down Esq., as a mark of esteem and respect for his ability and attainments by his teacher WJ Little'. (Courtesy of the Archives of the Royal London Hospital) — 21

The outpatient department at the London Hospital. The hospital served the poor of the East End. From *The Illustrated London News*, 1886 — 25

A signed copy of *Nature's Balance*, Langdon Down's prize essay, given to Mary Crellin 'with the best wishes of the author'. They married in 1860. (Courtesy of Mrs Patricia Langdon Down) — 26

The Royal Earlswood Asylum for Idiots, Redhill, Surrey, in 1880. (Courtesy of the Royal Earlswood Museum) — 32

Mary Langdon Down, photographed by her husband in 1865 — 44

An Earlswood dormitory, 1880. (Courtesy of the Royal Earlswood Museum) — 50

Mary with her first child, Everleigh, born in 1862 — 56

Everleigh, aged four years, dressed according to the prevailing custom. Boys did not wear trousers until at least the age of five years — 57

Lilian, the Langdon Downs' only daughter, aged two. Photographed by her father in the year she died — 58

The 'White House' in Hampton Wick, bought by the Langdon Downs in 1868. The name was changed to Normansfield — 78

The Rush mosaic, commissioned in 1893. The inscription reads: 'Blessing and honour and glory to be unto him that sitteth upon the throne'. The Langdon Down were devout Christians	80
The Normansfield boathouse, built in 1884 on the adjacent riverbank property purchased 11 years previously. The date of the photograph may be 1886, when the snowfall was so heavy that Normansfield had to purchase a snowplough	81
Langdon Down in court dress, 1887, when he gave the welcome address to the Prince and Princess of Wales at the opening of the London Hospital Nursing School. (Courtesy of the Archives of the Royal London Hospital)	91
Normansfield, showing the extensive accommodation which was added to increase the number of admissions. At one stage there were 156 patients in residence, plus the Langdon Down family and staff	97
Four Down's syndrome patients from the Earlswood series, photographed in 1865	101
Mary Langdon Down at the age of 55, wearing the diamond brooch her husband bought her for their silver wedding. He paid £45 for it (£2,700 today)	108
The Normansfield pageant for the Diamond Jubilee of Queen Victoria in 1897	112
The architect's drawing of the Normansfield theatre plan. Patients and staff were entertained in the theatre, commissioned in 1879. It has survived unchanged and, in its time, served both as an entertainment centre and a chapel. It is now classed as an historic building	116
The Normansfield theatre was host to the Genesta Amateur Dramatic Club, with which the Langdon Down family were associated. *The Illustrated Sporting and Dramatic News* of January 16th 1892 shows Miss M Bigwood in the role of Columbine. She later married Dr Percival Langdon Down	118
Every new member of staff was required to have musical or entertaining skills. Normansfield had an orchestra and a band made up of staff members. The photograph is from 1895	119

The Normansfield workshops. The nearest is the carpentry shop where Everleigh died; the furthest is the pharmacy. A photographic dark-room was partitioned off at the back of the pharmacy   124

The tombstone in the Nonconformist plot in Redhill cemetery, where Lilian was buried in 1865 and Everleigh in 1883. The inscription on the headstone describes the plot as the family grave of Langdon H and Mary Down, but only Lilian and Everleigh were buried there   126

Portrait of Langdon Down, painted by Sydney Hodges in 1883   133

Dr Reginald Langdon Down with his daughters Stella and Elspie. Stella married Russell Brain and became Lady Brain. Elspie was an artist. The only son was John, who had Down's syndrome   142

Reginald Langdon Down was the first to describe the pattern of creases in the palm in Down's syndrome patients. He drew this sketch in 1908   144

Dr Percival Langdon Down with his wife and children. His son, Norman, was to be the last Langdon Down superintendent of Normansfield, ending a family connection that had lasted for 102 years. The elder daughter, Molly, was also a doctor and worked in Normansfield   146

Mary A, the first Down's syndrome patient admitted to Normansfield, photographed when she was 19 and again when she was 55. She lived to the age of 58   151

Florence T, a Down's syndrome patient at Normansfield. Photographed in 1886 when she was seven and again in 1899 aged 20   155

James Henry Pullen, the *idiot savant* who designed the prize-winning exhibit for the Paris exhibition in 1867, dressed in the admiral's uniform which he accepted in return for not pursuing his plan to marry. He also designed a realistic model of the *Great Eastern*, a famous transatlantic vessel built by Brunel   168

Langdon Down's patient Elizabeth C. She has the short stature, severe obesity and characteristic facial appearance of Prader–Willi syndrome   171

Langdon Down with members of the British Medical Association in 1895 when he entertained 500 guests at Normansfield. He was founder President of the South Thames Branch   184

Langdon Down began to take clinical photographs in 1862. His first photograph of an Earlswood resident with Down's syndrome was this unnamed girl in the 1865 series. She was probably the first ever Down's syndrome patient to be photographed   190

An unnamed resident in the 1865 series, showing the small foreshortened head and what Langdon Down describes as a 'slightly apish nose', with deep-set eyes, possibly his Aztec prototype   192

The urn containing the ashes of John Langdon Down at the funeral service in the Normansfield theatre; his hospital gold medals are on a velvet cushion. Mary died five years later and their combined ashes were scattered in Normansfield   197

Table of Events

1828	John Langdon Down born in 27 Fore Street, Torpoint, the youngest of six children
1829	Baptized in Bethel Congregational chapel, Torpoint by the Reverend Joseph Sheppard
1833–42	Attended Dr Chubb's daughters' school and later Devonport Classical and Mathematical School
1842–46	Served as shop assistant in father's business. Chance encounter directed attention towards a medical career
1846	Apprenticed to Matthew Coleman MRCS at 265 Whitechapel Road, East London. Withdrew to study basic science at Pharmaceutical Society
1847	Passed minor and major examinations of Pharmaceutical Society with prize in organic chemistry. Returned to Torpoint and developed new pharmacy products for family business
1849	Returned to Pharmaceutical Society as laboratory assistant but became ill and returned again to Torpoint to convalesce
1852	Won prize essay competition on 'Nature's Balance', a religious theme. Essay published by Crockford's
1853	Death of his father. Decision to return to medicine. Enters London Hospital Medical School
1856	Passed MRCS examination in April and LSA in November. Awarded hospital gold medals in all clinical subjects and gold medal in materia medica, plus scholarship to University of London
1856–58	Resident accoucheur in obstetric department of London Hospital. Continued studies for University MB
1858	MB BCh with gold medals in physiology and comparative anatomy. Appointed medical superintendent at the Royal Earlswood Asylum for Idiots
1859	Passed Membership examination of Royal College of Physicians. Took MD in London University by examination
1859	Elected Assistant Physician at Royal London Hospital.
1860	Married Mary Crellin in Mare St Baptist Chapel
1861	First published paper on deficient corpus callosum
1862	Birth of first child, Everleigh. First patient photographs in Earlswood. *Lancet* paper on the mouth, a prelude to description of Down's syndrome
1863	Birth of Lilian, the only daughter
1864	Introductory address to medical students at London

	Hospital. Address to Pharmaceutical Society. Publications on scarlet fever and Prader–Willi syndrome
1865	Photographed over 200 residents in Earlswood. Death of Lilian
1866	Observations on an 'Ethnic Classification of Idiots' (description of Down's syndrome). London Hospital letter in support of admission of women to professions. Birth of Reginald
1867	*Lancet* paper on relationship between idiocy and tuberculosis
1868	Resigned Earlswood appointment. Commenced practice at 38 Welbeck Street and bought the White House, renamed Normansfield. First residents admitted. Birth of Percival
1869	Elected FRCP. Published four papers
1876	Published *The Education and Training of the Feeble in Mind*
1879	Normansfield theatre opened by Earl of Devon
1881	International Medical Congress reception at Normansfield. Purchased 81 Harley Street
1882	Chapter on Idiocy in Quain's *Medical Dictionary*
1883	Tragic death of Everleigh, aged 21
1884	Appointed Justice of the Peace. Normansfield boathouse built on River Thames
1885	Reginald's 21st birthday and Queen Victoria's Jubilee celebrations at Normansfield
1889	Elected as an Alderman for Middlesex. Percival's 21st birthday celebrations
1891	Congress of Hygiene reception for 500 guests. Genesta Amateur Dramatic Company started in Normansfield
1892	Reginald passed MB BCh examination
1893	Percival passed MB BCh. Arrangements for paying off last Normansfield mortgages
1895	Received 500 BMA guests at Normansfield
1896	Sudden death of John Langdon Down on 7th October. Cremation on 10th October, his wedding anniversary
1901	Death of Mary Langdon Down from influenza on 5th October
1961	Joint letter to *Lancet* from 25 genetic experts suggesting that the descriptive term 'Mongolism' be replaced by 'Down's syndrome'. Editor agrees
1966	World Health Organization adopts the eponymous term 'Down's syndrome'

Acknowledgements

Grateful thanks are expressed to the following: Mrs Patricia Langdon Down for easy access to family papers; Lord Christopher Brain for extensive genealogical studies, Mary Langdon Down's poem and crucial correspondence; Tony Langdon Down for the use of family photographs; Dr Michael Brain for Langdon Down's certificate of apprenticeship; The Lord Rix and the Friends of Normansfield for sponsorship of the Langdon Down Centenary meeting and the conservation of the Langdon Down photographs; Professor William Bynum of the Wellcome Institute for the History of Medicine for evaluating and amending the text; Paul Rowe for financial indices; Dr Nita Burnby, Editor of the *Pharmaceutical Historian*; Major Charles O'Leary, Honorary Archivist at the Worshipful Society for Apothecaries; Margaret Harcourt Williams, Archivist at the Royal College of Psychiatrists; Jonathan Evans, Archivist at the Royal London Hospital; Freda Knight of the East Surrey Hospital Library Service and Royal Earlswood Museum; Dr Frank James, of the Royal Institution of Great Britain; Professor Wolf Wolfensberger at Syracuse University and many others in the field of the history of medicine and of science.

Individual inquiries were answered by Julie Beckwith of the Royal College of Physicians Library; Professor C Breathnach of University College Dublin; Paul Cox in Milton Keynes; Heather Cadbury from the Teddington Area Reminiscence Group; Rev S Copson of the Baptist Historical Society; Professor M Esiri and Dr Brenda Hough at the Church of England Record Centre; Daphne Harkness of the London Diocesan Fund; Alisdair Hawkyard of the Harrow School Archives, Dr Milo Keynes in Cambridge; Pat and Freda Manning in the Torpoint Archives; Dr Stuart Mason in Essex; Rev WA McConnell of the Diocesan Council of Derry and Raphoe; Dr Sig Pueschel in Rochester; Dr Norbert Pies of Ersfstadt-Lechenich; Dr Caroline Reid of the Royal Pharmaceutical Society Museum; Dr RP Snaith of the University of Leeds; Dr Richard Shepherd at St George's Hospital; Dr Alex Sakula in Reigate; June Sampson of the *Surrey Comet*; Dr D Wright of the University of Nottingham; Rev Philip Warner of Teddington; Dr Richard Wilson in Kingston-upon-Thames and Professor W Wolfensberger of Syracuse University.

The following archives departments contributed generously to the background research: the Metropolitan London Records Office, Surrey Record Office, Royal Society of Medicine, Ashmolean Museum Oxford, Chatsworth House Devonshire Collections, Powderham Castle Archives, Guildhall Library, Stratford Museum and Archives, University of London Library, Wellcome Institute for the History of Medicine, BMA Archives, the Royal College of Physicians, the Royal College of Psychiatrists, the Royal College of Physicians of Ireland and the Medical Society of London. The resources of the BMA library were also used extensively. Ray Lunnon, the Curator of the Great Ormond Street Hospital Archives department, provided historical photographic data and, with Ken Simmons, Archival Photographer to the Surrey Record Office, catalogued and conserved the Langdon Down photographs. Steve Curran facilitated the use of Normansfield records. Maureen Ryan patiently typed the initial drafts and Lydia Nicholls edited the manuscript for the Royal Society of Medicine Press with tolerant professionalism.

To these and to many others the author expresses heartfelt thanks.

Foreword

John Langdon Down has suffered all three of the fates which can befall a pioneer in an area of work about which there are strong opinions, not always accompanied by close familarity. He has been ignored, sanctified and vilified. He was a man of his time, with great insight compared to many of his contemporaries, but with some of the inevitable limitations that are to be expected when so much of the knowledge and the means of acquiring knowledge – which we now take for granted – were simply not available.

He was, supremely, someone who took both the trouble to observe and made the effort to care. He did it for people with learning disability who, then as now, are not always seen by everyone as being worth that trouble and effort. A few of his observations led to false conclusions and some of his methods of providing care were – with the wisdom born of a century of hindsight and further evidence – unhelpful, although seldom worse than no care at all.

I like a man who looks closely, asks questions, develops conclusions, tries things out and revises conclusions in the light of further evidence. We call such people scientists. I like men who recognize in others the common ground of shared humanity; who act on the basis of that shared humanity and do what they can to spread a little happiness to those without much going for them. I like men who value what others have to offer, who encourage those gifts and give them opportunity and credit. I like men who, blessed with a talented and competent wife, enter into an equal partnership with that wife. I like John Langdon Down.

Needless to say I never met him but I entered, in a manner of speaking, into the inheritance left by him and his wife in Normansfield Hospital; my wife and I have reason to be grateful that Normansfield was there when our daughter needed it. Its successor services were also there when the time came for Shelley to move on to a more normal way of life in the local community.

John Langdon Down has become part of the history of treatment, care and support for people with learning disabilities – a history with its fair share of faults, but also much that is good. There are many points from which we can learn, more than a hundred years after his death, from his life as depicted in this extensive biography. I would list in particular: looking at the whole person and not just the learning disability; maintaining optimism about every person's ability to move forward (however modest their predicted achievements); trying to offer people things that are likely to give them pleasure (always provided that they are not even more likely to do them harm) and paying attention to the inner person, including body and spirit.

I would, however, put at the top of my list willingness to learn – which often means learning and relearning. It is so easy for all of us to convince ourselves that what we are doing is right, to the extent of refusing to notice the evidence against it. In relation to the condition which has come to be associated most closely with John Langdon Down, namely Down's syndrome (or as some would have it Down syndrome), he seems to have been wiser than some of his contemporaries in separating out a physical appearance which might loosely be described as 'Mongoloid' from the ethnic theories that sprang from that observation. In other words, he carried on thinking where others stopped.

It is good to think that, as the terminology of mental retardation, mental subnormality, mental handicap, learning disability and intellectual disability comes and goes, we are likely to keep 'Down's syndrome' as both non-offensive language and a tribute to a great man. At risk of stirring a much wider debate, may I add that our society would be a great deal poorer if Dr Langdon Down – and those named after him – had never been born. Together, they have challenged many long-held myths and misunderstandings. We owe them a debt which we must repay.

The Lord Rix CBE DL
Chairman, Friends of Normansfield
Chairman, Mencap
August, 1998

Introduction

The life of John Langdon Down is the story of a man who climbed from almost the lowest rung to the highest reach of the social ladder. His life was extraordinary. He was taken from school at the age of 14 to work in the family grocery business. Within the business there was a pharmacy department; he went on to qualify as a pharmacist and to develop a succesful range of new products. When he later entered the London Hospital Medical School he showed brilliant promise and, immediately after taking his University degree, he became Medical Superintendent of the Royal Earlswood Asylum for Idiots. It was here that he made the observation that was to make him posthumously famous – the identification of the special characteristics of what he called Mongolian idiocy, now called Down's syndrome. He was one of the famous medical men in a golden age of London medicine. Apart from Down's syndrome he was also the first to describe another serious medical condition, now called Prader–Willi syndrome.

He was an outstanding campaigner for better care for people with learning disability and, in Normansfield, his own private training institute, he lived under the same roof as his patients. He saw the disabled banished to the servants' quarters at home and wanted to give them a better life. He was among the first to identify the value of clinical photography and his surviving archive of patients' clinical photographs is the biggest collection in either the US or UK. Perhaps his life story has never been written because he was such a model of earnest propriety; the smooth tenor of his family life was interrupted only by the sad deaths of his first two children and the story of how they died has never been told. He had a natural empathy with handicapped children. Charles Buxton MP called him 'the right man in the right place' and described how children followed him like a Pied Piper 'taking his hand and evincing their unfeigned delight in his presence'[1].

The Normansfield account books show how he gradually built up the 43 acre estate in suburban London and how, from having no capital, he became one of London's wealthiest doctors. He was ahead of his time in approving of the advancement of women in medicine, the law and the church and was associated with the campaign to give women the right to vote. His own marriage to Mary Crellin was one of devoted loyalty and, when she died, their ashes were scattered together in the grounds of Normansfield, their hospital and home. His life was one of Christian rectitude and his motivation came from a simple faith which he carried with him to his death. The Langdon Downs survived the sad deaths of two of their four children, but lived to see their two surviving sons well-established in the medical profession. The story of John Langdon Down is one of great human interest and it is a matter of regret that his great contributions to medicine and society have never been fully recognized.

Reference
1   Surrey Records Office. SRO 392/1/2/1. Annual Report, 1864. F255.

Chapter 1

Early Life

Down's syndrome was first recognized by John Langdon Down in 1866. He was one of the outstanding clinicians of his time and, in due course, he became both rich and famous – a figure of society, Justice of the Peace, alderman of Middlesex and treasurer of the ancient Guild of Broderers. When he died in November 1896 his funeral ceremonies were marked by pomp and dignity. He was later commemorated by the naming of two streets after him, Down Street in Teddington and Langdon Down Way in his native Torpoint; he had travelled a long way from his humble early days.

He was born in 1828, the youngest of six children. The family lived at 27 Fore Street in Torpoint where, from 1815, his father owned a shop over which the family lived. Joseph Almond Down is listed in local records as 'a druggist, grocer and linen draper', in a business called Down & Son[1]. The son was Richard, born in 1810. As the eldest he exerted a great deal of influence in family affairs and John came to resent the extent to which his life was controlled by his older brother. Number 27 was a small house and, even when it was combined with Number 26 to extend the business, the accommodation was limited.

Joseph Almond Down was born in Hackney, London. He had a chequered career, involving an apprenticeship to a druggist followed by three business failures. The knowledge of his father's failures left John Langdon Down with an anxiety about bankruptcy and, in later life, when well-established, he frequently referred to scientific knowledge as an asset which could never be affected by insolvency. Joseph probably never completed any formal professional apprenticeship. When the Pharmaceutical Society was formed in 1841, he did not take the opportunity of registering, although, at that time, he could have become a member without taking an entrance examination. His business failures all happened before Langdon Down was born, but his mother may have told him about them when he was a child. He was very close to her and she may have confided in him about the worries and indignities she had endured.

The business failures of Joseph Almond Down may have been a symptom of a serious personal problem. When he died in 1853 his death certificate listed the causes of death as sub-acute gout (podagra), inflammation of the liver and cerebral congestion. The listed contributory causes to his death suggest that he drank to excess, at least on occasion. Langdon Down was a very caring person and in his father's last years he may have been the one to be called when the drinking got out of hand. He was recalled to Torpoint many times because of filial duty, but it was probably the health of his father and not the health of the business that brought him back[2].

Throughout his medical career Langdon Down referred many times to the dangers of excessive drinking. Temperance was heavily promoted in Cornwall after the visits of John Wesley but Langdon Down may have learned his lesson a hard way. The death certificate of Joseph Almond Down lists John Langdon as being present at the time of his death. Later in life, clinical notes refer frequently to Langdon Down being in attendance at patients' deathbeds and his father's death may have been the first to test his compassion and composure. Langdon Down's concern about the ill-effects of alcohol were later reinforced when his brother, Kelland, also developed a drink problem. Kelland left the family business in 1850 and ended up in the workhouse in Liverpool in debt and misery, appealing for money and threatening to set out to walk to London to get it from his family.

After his business failures, fortune finally favoured Joseph Almond in his new venture in Torpoint. In this business he had, for the first time, the advantage of family support. The grocery store gave an opportunity for his wife Hannah to show her worth and the family certainly gave her credit for the success of the enterprise. When Langdon Down was 11 he and his mother rode out on horseback to visit her agents and rode 14 miles in a day.

Richard, 18 years older than John, was also a good businessman and ultimately took over and diversified the business. This was the time when activities in the retail trade were separated by hazy boundaries; chemists and druggists sold groceries and grocers sold drugs. Apothecaries, who compounded medicines on prescription, also gave medical advice. Richard had gone to London in 1831 for training in the drugs business. Unpublished family correspondence points to his having 'engaged himself to a gentleman who had an open surgery in connection with his business as an apothecary'. He probably stayed in London for just one year.

Neither Joseph Almond Down nor his son Richard appear on the register of the Worshipful Society of Apothecaries and Joseph Almond Down described himself as a grocer in the census form for 1841. He apparently did not lay claim to the title of apothecary during his working life, although the fact that he was partially engaged in the drug trade came to be of importance later when John Langdon Down took his first basic medical qualification, the certificate of the Worshipful Society of Apothecaries, in 1856.

He had started at the local school at the age of five, moving at eight to a boys school and again at 11 to the Devonport Classical and

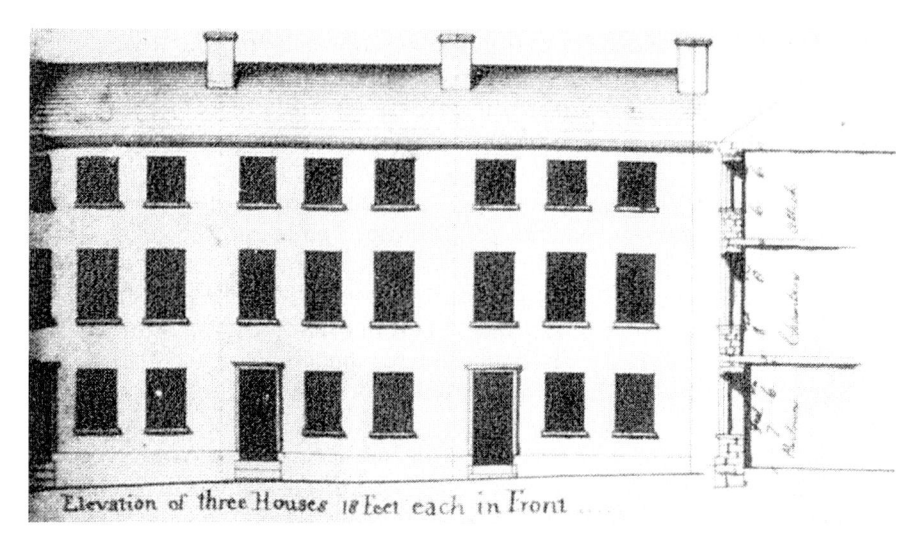

Plan of Torpoint houses. All were built to the same design in narrow streets.

Mathematical School where he spent his last three years. Leaving school as he did at an early age, he never had an opportunity of learning Latin and Greek. This was to be a disadvantage to him when he later applied to enter medical school. Entrance scholarships included Latin and Greek as examination subjects and so he was debarred.

The Down family considered themselves to be among the poor in the town and even in 1871 Richard, writing to the Secretary of State concerning the need for a water supply wrote 'we, the Poor Inhabitants of this Town, most humbly pray that you will please take into consideration that we are dreadfully in want of a supply of water in the Town... we have [to]... go to the Town well which is in the lower part of the Town and is only approachable by descending about 30 steps to get at the water for the supply of the whole of the poor of the Town. On each side of this well runs the common sewer which makes the water very unhealthy for us poor people'[3].

At least the Downs did not have to use the common sewer; the Torpoint housing plan shows that the houses in Fore Street had outside privies. However poor water supply led to two outbreaks of cholera, in 1832 and 1849. There were 38 deaths, but the Down family escaped. During the second epidemic it was recognized that the contaminated water supply was a crucial factor. Water was shipped into the town from the naval shipyard by tanker as an emergency measure, but it was not until 1884 that the water supply and drainage system were put in order.

The Down family business was open between 7 am and 9 pm so, early in life, John Langdon Down became conditioned to hard work and long working hours. In 1841 the census shows there were four live-in employees[4]. Perhaps the wages of staff seemed to be an excessive burden and young John was seen as someone who could earn his keep. In any event he was taken out of school at the age of 14 to work behind the counter.

The Downs faced competition from two other grocers in Torpoint, but the business went from strength to strength and, by 1854, it became necessary to rent an unoccupied varnish house as additional storage space. The expanding business required more staff and, in 1851, the census report showed that there were 11 people – both family and staff – living in the upstairs accommodation. These included Hannah who, with her husband, had moved out in 1843 when Richard married Susan Durant, but moved back in again later at the time of the census. There were three live-in assistants, two nieces and two house servants, in addition to Richard's three children and, of course, his brother John. Conditions must have been very crowded. John was by now a paid full-time employee, but remained under great pressure to become a permanent member of staff. An unpublished letter to his brother-in-law, Philip Crellin, tells how he hated the retail business, apart from the pharmaceutical side[5].

The Torpoint experience was to stand John Langdon Down in good stead; he had, in his father's shop, been introduced to the problems of those who were sick but too poor to afford a doctor's fee. Patients came to the grocer-chemist for treatment. He learned early in life to care for people, whom later in his career he would be expected to cure. He was not destined to spend his life in a grocer's apron.

After the death of John Langdon Down, his family, who were by then rich and famous, showed themselves to be somewhat sensitive about his humble beginnings. An imaginative family tree, giving a line of descent from the Protestant Bishop of Derry was drawn up. Unfortunately, *Crockford's Clerical Directory* does not list any Bishop Down and the family tree, now extensively researched, has still not bridged the gap in the line of descent.

John Langdon Down's birth certificate lists his full name as John Langdon Haydon Down. The Langdon family was an old established one and it can be traced at Braunton in Devon back to the 16th century. Langdon Down's maternal grandmother was Jane Langdon and he always signed himself as John Langdon Down. The Haydon name can be traced to the 17th century and one branch of the family owned substantial estates, but a direct connection to the Langdon Down family has not been traced. John Langdon Down's family tree was formidable, but less distinguished than was claimed after his death.

The Langdon Down family were devoutly religious. Joseph Almond Down, his father, was one of the first subscribers to the original lease of the Congregational Chapel in 1812[6], where John Langdon Down was baptized. The strong religious convictions of the family may have come down from his grandfather, Joseph

Kelland Down who, on 26 August, 1795, perhaps feeling that his religious affairs were in disarray, had three of his children baptized on the same day, suggesting a new burst of religious activity. Throughout Langdon Down's childhood and youth the family maintained a strong connection with the Congregational Church in Torpoint and his brother Richard, in particular, was heavily involved. When Richard married in 1843, his wife moved into the Fore Street family home. Joseph Almond Down and Hannah moved out and Richard became the effective head of the business. The 15-year-old John now found himself employed by his older brother. He spent the next four years learning the trade of grocer and purveyor of proprietary medicines.

References

1 *Pigot's Commercial Directory of 1830.*
2 Obituary. *BMJ* 1896; **2**: 1170–1.
3 Harris G, Harris FL. *The Making of a Cornish Town.* Penzance: Herdland Publishers, 1976: 100.
4 Census return, 1841. Parish of St Antony CS41/2.
5 Unpublished correspondence, courtesy of Lord Christopher Brain.
6 C/54/9/9752. Public Records Office.

Chapter 2

The Pharmaceutical Chemist

In 1846 an event occurred which was to change John Langdon Down's life. In a public address, at the opening of major extensions in Normansfield in 1879 he recorded what had happened:

> In a remote part of the country on an alfresco picnic... driven by stress of weather into a cottage on the coast, I was brought into contact with a feeble minded girl, who waited on our party and for whom the question haunted me – could nothing for her be done? I had then not entered on a medical student's career, but ever and anon the remembrance of that hapless girl presented itself to me and I longed to do something for her kind[1].

He had also seen the very poor lifestyle of two families of children with learning disabilities in Torpoint. One family was rich, the other poor; conditions were bad for both[2].

He lacked advice on how to bring his dream to fulfilment and had to contend with the opposition of his directive older brother. Years later, in his paper on the obstetrical aspects of idiocy, he writes; 'one very interesting and important point suggested by my enquiries is that of primogeniture. We know how much our political system hangs on the laws of primogeniture, how the first born inherits property and inherits the power to rule over his fellows and how much our whole social structure is based thereon'[3]. His brother was indeed to inherit the business but, above all else, to exercise the authority of the head of the family. Unfortunately Joseph Almond Down's will cannot be traced, owing to the loss of records during the second world war. He may of course have left no will, and it may not have been necessary for him to write one as Richard was already designated as the only partner in Down and Son. There was an age gap of 18 years between the brothers and John never became an equal partner with Richard in the business.

John Langdon Down's first faltering step towards medicine was taken in 1846. There was no family tradition of medical practice on which he could draw. It may indeed have been a part of a business master-plan to graft a fully-fledged apothecary's practice on to the grocery/pharmacy. He went to London and was apprenticed to Matthew Coleman at 265 Whitechapel Rd. The new apprentice was taught to extract teeth, apply leeches, let blood and apply blisters; apothecaries did all of this and compounded medicines. Langdon Down bought the published London University past examination papers from the year 1841 and the standards alarmed him; he had taught himself some science but needed to learn far more if he was to progress in medicine.

The Pharmaceutical Society had, he discovered, put in place a very good course for aspiring pharmaceutical chemists. He was later to acknowledge that chemistry was better taught there than anywhere else in London, and that medical students could never learn the amount of botany and materia medica taught to pharmacists[4]. If he took this course he would enter medical school with a very good basic knowledge, not only of physics and chemistry, but also botany and materia medica. If he returned to Torpoint he might have a dual role, combining pharmacy with medicine.

The fee for the year-long course in the Pharmaceutical Society was £38 which, presumably, his family paid. He may have lived in the Pharmaceutical Society premises in 17 Bloomsbury Square; the records of the Pharmaceutical Society in the following years frequently give this as an address for some students, who may have lodged in the attic rooms. It is perhaps more likely however that he lodged with Dr Coleman.

His father's health was failing. The business was expanding but was also seen to have a potential for upgrading in the pharmacy department and his brother Richard had limited experience of the drug business. There was at that time a great deal of public discussion concerning the control of the pharmaceutical profession and examination and registration of pharmaceutical chemists was on the horizon. To have a properly qualified pharmaceutical chemist in the business might, in the future, become increasingly important. The family pressures to settle in Torpoint were intense and his name was even entered jointly with that of his father in the lease of a property in Torpoint Field[5]. There were family expectations that he would return to Torpoint, settle there and work for, or with, his brother. The business came first and he could serve it as well if he trained as a pharmacist as he could if he became an apothecary, but in a much shorter time.

Only the élite of the pharmaceutical profession took the Pharmaceutical Society course. Only 80 students were registered out of approximately 3000 pharmaceutical trainees in the UK[6] and only 31 of the 80 students to be admitted could be accommodated in the teaching laboratories. Down was one of the lucky ones.

The Pharmaceutical Society was working to elevate the trade of chemist and druggist to the profession of pharmaceutical chemist. This was to be a long process and it was not until 1858 that it became necessary to become a member of the Pharmaceutical Society in order to practice as a pharmaceutical chemist. The Pharmaceutical Society teachers were men of great distinction. Apart from Theophilus Redwood who taught chemistry and pharmacy, Anthony Todd Thompson taught botany and Jonathon

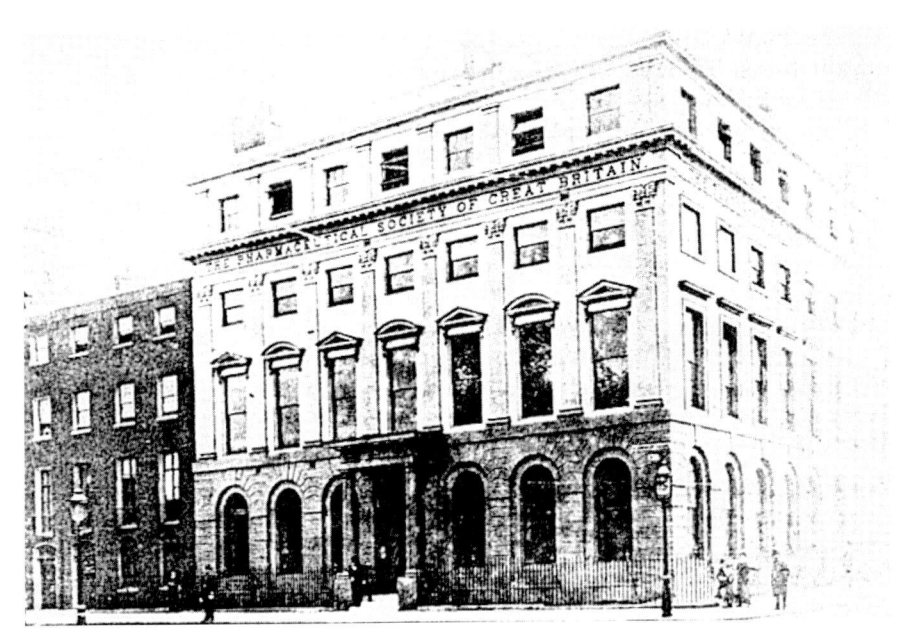

The Pharmaceutical Society, 1845.

Pereira materia medica. Physics had also been taught initially by Theophilus Redwood, who appears to have been able to turn his hand to any subject. He was later to take over chemistry from Dr George Fownes. Langdon Down won the prize in organic chemistry, his first major academic distinction, in 1849. He passed the two examinations of the Society, the Minor and Major, in quick succession in June and July of the same year. He clearly had reservations about joining the business of Down & Son and never registered as a member of the Pharmaceutical Society.

One month after John Langdon Down had taken his final examination, his brother Richard was admitted a member of the Society. He had not taken any examinations but, as the head of an existing business, was entitled to be admitted on that basis. It is likely that Joseph Almond Down was by then in failing health. Before he died he effectively retired, leaving Richard in charge and putting him in the position of being able to register. John's newly acquired qualification put the business, now known as Down Brothers, in an unassailable position with the addition of a qualified pharmaceutical chemist. The Down brothers, who were the registered owners of the business were Richard and Kelland, the second eldest son. The evolution of registration for pharmaceutical chemists was gradual. Even up to 1868 it was possible for a pharmaceutical chemist who had not taken examinations to become a registered member of the Pharmaceutical Society on the affidavit of a doctor or magistrate confirming that he had been in the business of chemist and druggist.

Pharmacists and druggists, particularly in working class areas, often practised illegally as apothecaries, although The Worshipful Society of Apothecaries monitored practice carefully. Everything was changing however and the 1815 Apothecaries Act made it clear that, in future, candidates should be examined in the science and practice of medicine; apprenticeship alone would no longer suffice. At the same time lines of demarcation between medicine and pharmacy were becoming clearer. The outcome of his Royal Pharmaceutical Society training was that John Langdon Down became a qualified pharmaceutical chemist, though he remained unregistered. He did not lend his name to the family business although, with his new found knowledge, he was able to be of practical assistance. He helped Richard to move quickly into a phase of drug manufacture and formulation and the pharmacy retail business expanded greatly.

The training for the difficult examinations of the Royal Pharmaceutical Society would have prepared him for when he later became a medical student. There was great emphasis placed on practical laboratory training in the Royal Pharmaceutical Society and each student had to buy 30 items of laboratory equipment. This intensive laboratory experience could not but increase John Langdon Down's powers of observation, manual dexterity and range of interests. Langdon Down retained a connection with the Royal Pharmaceutical Society throughout his lifetime and his obituary in the *Pharmaceutical Journal* records that he was a warm friend of the Society and that he was enthusiastically appreciative of the benefit he had derived from the Society's School[8]. He gave the opening address at the inauguration of the academic year in the Royal Pharmaceutical Society on 6 October, 1888 and, in his opening remarks, said: '...my affections have been entwined from the very commencement of your Society around the noble and successful efforts to advance pharmacy in Great Britain and from the recollection that it was within the walls of this building that I received, some 37 years since, my first scientific impulses and my earliest scientific training'[4].

John Langdon Down returned to Torpoint. His return and the rapid admission of his brother Richard to membership of the Pharmaceutical Society revolutionized the family business. In 1849 his mentor, Theophilus Redwood, published as co-author a translation of a textbook produced by Francis Mohr of Coblenz on *Practical Pharmacy: The Arrangements, Apparatus and Manipulations of the Pharmaceutical Shop and Laboratory*[7]. Langdon Down was at the Royal Pharmaceutical Society while this book was being completed and would have had ample opportunity of profiting from Redwood's involvement while he had the book in hand. The book was well-illustrated and provided all the necessary information for the setting up of a small manufacturing process. It had 400 woodcuts and the aspiring manufacturer was taken step-by-step through the procedure for the bulk production of medications.

Langdon Down masterminded the production of new products which were widely advertised and six of the Down advertising flyers have survived. These covered diarrhoea, indigestion, catarrh, cough, temperature and neuralgia. The Down pharmacy now marketed a complete range of pharmaceutical products. Down's pectoral cough lozenges, 'prepared only by RH Down, member of the Pharmaceutical Society', were sold at 7½ d per box and they could be sent by post for 9d. A diarrhoea mixture, 'prepared from an improvement on the form supplied by the Board of Health during a cholera epidemic in 1849' soon followed. The recent experience of cholera in Torpoint clearly generated a sense of urgency. The flyer was headed 'Advice Gratis, which it would be unwise to neglect'. In addition there was Down's

Advice Gratis

WHICH IT WOULD BE VERY UNWISE TO NEGLECT.

Persons suffering from an attack of Diarrhœa, should at once procure a Bottle of

DIARRHŒA MIXTURE

Prepared from an improvement on the form supplied by the Board of Health during the Cholera of 1849, since which it has been taken by thousands of persons with almost unvarying success. No family should be without it; in nine cases out of ten no other Medicine will be required, and in most cases Two Doses will effect a cure.

Sold in Bottles at 8d. each, or double the size at 1/2 by

R. H. DOWN, M.P.S.,
DISPENSING CHEMIST,
TORPOINT.

Advertising flyer for Richard Down's diarrhoea mixture.

volatile liniment, his celebrated pearl ointment for wounds and all kinds of disease of the skin, 'whose efficacy has been proved by thousands', and quinine wine, recommended for neuralgia, chronic and pulmonary catarrh, scrofulous conditions of the system and chronic diarrhoea.

Toilet preparations were also heavily advertised. There was Down's Lemon Juice and Glycerine and Down's Rose Dentifrice contained a vegetable powder to impart an aromatic fragrance to the breath. It whitened the teeth, preserved the enamel, and by its antiseptic properties arrested and eventually prevented decay. There was Down's Celebrated Lavender Water and Down's Vaseline Pomade, a new remedy for weak or thin hair, which stimulated the roots of the hair, removed scurf and rendered the hair soft and glossy. Down Brothers also sold pure carbolic acid, coal tar and other fancy soaps and hair, tooth and nail brushes.

John Langdon Down was employed by his brother at a salary of £50 per annum and the firm clearly got value for money in terms of his newly-acquired technical knowledge. In addition Jonathon Pereira, who had taught Langdon Down materia medica, was one of the greatest contemporary experts on the properties of drugs and their uses. He was the author of *Selectio Ex Praescriptis*, a standard reference book on medication, first published in 1837 and running to eight editions[9]. Langdon Down had acquired expert knowledge of drug formulation; the new products which were launched under the name of Richard Down, MPS and which were to bring fame and fortune to the pharmacy were the result of Langdon Down's special training.

Langdon Down may also have come to the assistance of his other brother Henry. Henry had a business in Woburn, described as that of chemist, druggist and grocer. The business was later to specialize in agrichemicals – 'Ossiline' for horses' joints and 'The Farmer's Friend' for the protection of wheat from smut were widely advertised. The timing of the emergence of these new manufactured products suggests that Langdon Down may have helped to formulate them; alternatively, he had the necessary training to analyse and copy a rival product. The two branches of the family maintained close contact; many years later Henry Down's son, also Henry, attended the 21st birthday celebration of Langdon Down's son, Percival. When Henry got pneumonia in 1891 Langdon Down set out by special train to Woburn to consult with Mr Lucas, his surgeon, but Henry died before his brother arrived.

Jonathon Pereira became a lifelong friend and his advice was undoubtedly of great value to John Langdon Down when he later switched careers from pharmacy to medicine, as Pereira had done. He started his professional life by serving as an apprentice to an apothecary and ended up in the London Hospital, where he was appointed Lecturer in Chemistry and, later, Assistant Physician.

This upward movement must have influenced Langdon Down, who was to follow a similar path.

When John Langdon Down's obituaries came to be written the family pride of the Langdon Downs and their sensitivity concerning John Langdon Down's humble origins led them to over-emphasize the importance of his scientific career before he studied medicine. He was listed in two obituaries as having assisted Faraday – the discoverer of electro-magnetism – in his experiments, which implied that he was an important collaborator[10,11]. Faraday however kept a diary of his experiments and only one of them was conducted in the laboratory of the Pharmaceutical Society in 1850[12]. Langdon Down may have seen this experiment, but a newly graduated laboratory assistant can scarcely have had any significant role and Faraday never referred to any contact with Langdon Down in subsequent correspondence.

With his Pharmaceutical Society examinations to his credit Langdon Down busied himself in Torpoint with the new pharmacy products. A new career beckoned however; when he had been at home for just one year he was offered an appointment as a laboratory assistant to work for Professor Redwood. There is no record in the Royal Pharmaceutical Society of the nature of this appointment but, in the light of his limited experience, it probably involved mainly supervision of students' laboratory bench work. He clearly did well and at the dinner of the School of the Pharmacy held in the London Tavern on 17 July, 1848, Professor Redwood referred to him, together with his fellow assistant Mr Braithwaite: 'It is a source of much gratification to those connected with the management of the School to find young men who have been pupils in the school becoming, in their turn, efficient ministers of instruction...'[13]. Langdon Down and Theophilus Redwood had a lot in common. In religion both were Nonconformists. They had had experience in the retail trade and had left school early to work in a family retail business and both were men of exceptional talent and industry who lived to see their efforts rewarded.

References

1 *Christian Union*, 27 June 1879.
2 Normansfield. *Medical Times*, 28 June 1879.
3 Down JLD. On the obstetrical aspects of idiocy. In: *Mental Affections of Childhood*. London: Churchill, 1887.
4 Down JLD. Inaugural Address. *Pharmaceutical Journal* 1880; **49**: 289–93.
5 Cornwall County Records Office, AD/829-260.
6 Holloway SWF. *Royal Pharmaceutical Society of Great Britain 1841–91*. London: Pharmaceutical Press, 1991.

7   Redwood T. *Practical Pharmacy*. London: Taylor Walton & Maberly, 1849.
8   Obituary. *Pharm J* 1896; **57**: 326–30.
9   Pereira J. *Selectio Ex Praescriptis*, 1837.
10 Obituary. *BMJ* 1896; **2**: 1170–1.
11 Obituary. *Lancet* 1896; **2**: 11704–5.
12 *Faraday's Diary*. G Bell & Sons, 1934: 287.
13 Annual Dinner Report. *Pharm J* 1849; **50**: 9,61.

------- Chapter 3 -------

Return to Torpoint

Langdon Down's appointment as a laboratory assistant was not to last. There was a conflict between the facts as set out in the *BMJ* and the *Lancet* obituaries[1,2] as to why he left his post in the Pharmaceutical Society; the *BMJ* stated that he was urgently summoned home, the *Lancet* that he left because his health broke down. The latter appears to fit the facts. In a letter to his brother-in-law Philip Crellin, on 2nd May 1853 he wrote:

> I have for some time decided with the concurrence of friends here to leave Torpoint this autumn. My principal reason for coming here, restoration of my health, has been in great measure effected, and the looking forward to a perpetual residence here is out of the question. The drug business has attained its maximum extent (doubled), and the other departments I detest, partly from not understanding them[3].

There may have been an element of truth in both obituaries, as his father's health was poor and, from then until 1853, Langdon Down was probably in effect his counsellor, attendant in times of crisis and main psychological support.

The nature of the illness from which Langdon Down suffered has never been clarified. Unpublished family correspondence refers to his suffering from the effects of inhaling noxious vapours, implying that he had developed a troublesome cough and also that he had lost 17 pounds in weight. The combination of weight loss and a persistent cough would seem to fit with a diagnosis of tuberculosis, as would the history of spontaneous recovery over a period of three years, during which he rested, rode across the moors, walked and engaging in 'health seeking'.

He made a good recovery and, during his convalescence, continued to help in the business; he was still paid £50 a year by his brother. He also lectured at the Mechanics Institutes at Devonport, Looe, Liskeard and Torpoint. His greatest accomplishment however, was his prize essay, read at the Stonehouse Institute in the autumn of 1852. This was entitled 'Nature's Balance'[4] with the theme of 'the wisdom and beneficence of the Creator as displayed in the compensation between the animal and vegetable kingdoms'. The essay was to be published by Crockford's, the publishers of the *Church of England Ecclesiastical Directory* and was first delivered publicly at the

Stonehouse Institution. It was published in 1853. He dedicated the published essay to Theophilus Redwood, Professor of Chemistry and Pharmacy to the Pharmaceutical Society of Great Britain as a token of esteem and regard by his late pupil and assistant.

The rather clumsy title was copied from the title of an endowment in the Royal Society set up in 1830 by the Earl of Bridgewater. The endowment of £8000 to the Royal Society was to be paid to persons nominated by the President of the Society to write, publish and print 1000 copies of an essay to be entitled: 'On the power, wisdom and goodness of God as manifest in the Creation'. The object of the endowment was clearly to emphasize the role of the Almighty Creator at a time when the theory of evolution might have been perceived to come in conflict with the established ideas concerning the creation of the world and of vegetable, animal and human life. In the Royal Society the nominated participants were high ranking ecclesiastics and philosophers. It was probably no coincidence that the President of the Stonehouse Institute selected the same topic for the prize essay. The essay was to be of a convenient length for a public reading at the end of the winter session. Langdon Down undoubtedly acquitted himself well. He was an eloquent speaker and in later life was distinguished for his formal oratory.

He introduced the essay with a disclaimer that neither the substance nor the argument would present anything new to the scientifically informed. He had the common touch and spoke to the interested amateurs without condescension. Having to crystallize his thoughts in writing led him to define his position as a man, a scientist in the making and a Christian. In his concluding paragraph he refers to the pre-eminence in creation of the human soul: 'We have made use of the light that chemistry emits in surveying the processes of organisation; but it would be wrong to infer that it is other than subordinate to that potent principle, call it what we please, that was, according to the Holy Record, breathed into the nostrils of our first parent when he became a living soul'[4].

His prize-winning essay spoke of the accumulated labours of the astronomer providing a boundless view of the omnipotence of God. He referred poetically to the fossils found by geologists, proclaiming from their rocky home in audible voices the eternity of Almighty God. He went on to paint on a broad canvas the structure and function of lower life forms, outlining the difference between the beautiful but disorganized symmetry of mineral crystals and the contrasting organization of cell tissues. He dealt with the way which cells maintain vital activity and the balance between the accumulation of new tissues and the disintegration of old tissues. As in geology and astronomy, he referred to leading facts of chemistry to show the admirable arrangement of the Divine Intelligence and how it could teach man in his pride that he should be humble in the face of his Creator. Throughout his life he lived and spoke of living in the presence of God.

The differentiation of forms of life fascinated him and he wondered at the ordering of nature. He speculated on the versatility of plants and how, using a similar apparatus of cells and tubes, one plant could produce quinine for the relief of fever and another a deadly output of strychnine. He saw a continuity between the animal and vegetable species and pointed out that sponges showed characteristics of both and bridged the gap. He saw the role of plants in removing carbon dioxide as protecting the animal world from gaseous intoxication.

This perception of even the lowest forms of life as mirroring the facets of divine perfection was the underlying basis of his acceptance of people with disability, reflecting that in each there was some aspect, or hope, of perfection. The graded merging of species and sophistication which he described was also the basis for his concept of upward progression of ability from low starting levels to higher peaks of accomplishment. At an early age he had formulated the philosophy and mode of thought which was to sustain his professional work.

References

1 Obituary. *BMJ* 1896; **2**: 1170–1.
2 Obituary. *Lancet* 1896; **2**: 1104–5.
3 Unpublished correspondence, courtesy of Lord Christopher Brain.
4 Down JL. *Nature's Balance*. Crockford's, 1852.

Chapter 4

To Medical School

At home again in Torpoint, medicine beckoned once more. His father, already retired, signed a new apprentice's indenture which entitled Langdon Down to claim the role of apothecary in training (Appendix 1). His apprenticeship to Dr Coleman had by then lapsed. When his father died, in 1853, Langdon Down took stock of his future. In his letter to his brother-in-law, Philip Crellin, on 2nd May[1] he discoursed at length about his choice of career. One thing was certain – he was determined not to continue in the family business. The two options in his mind were medicine, which he put first, and science. Medicine was his first choice but in real terms he saw that he could not afford it. He wrote of entering one of the cheaper hospitals for three years and of giving his services as a dispenser to some surgeon in return for his board. He also hoped that in medical school his knowledge of the several branches of study would place him at an advantage in prize contests and would procure for him some public appointment in due course. Out of the £50 per year which had come to him from his brother he had managed to save £100. In one year he had spent only £15 on clothes and everything else that he bought. He reckoned that, as the fees for full attendance at the Middlesex Hospital together with the lectures were £75, he could manage independently of anyone, but there remained the problem of his board and lodging.

His second choice was to go to Giessen University in Germany to study chemistry under Professor Liebig; in case this option had to be exercised he had studied German during the winter. He foresaw this alternative as giving an opening in translating German scientific works into English, emulating his mentor Theophilus Redwood, or of becoming involved in academic chemistry or manufacturing. His choice of Giessen was not accidental. Jacob Bell, the driving force behind the institution of the Royal Pharmaceutical Society, and a wealthy dispensing chemist, entertained hospitably at his address at 338 Oxford Street. Redwood was a frequent guest at his house and he assisted Bell in editing the *Pharmaceutical Transactions*. Liebig and Redwood were good friends and Liebig later masterminded the award of a Giessen University PhD to Redwood. Moving as he did in the inner circles of the advancing pharmaceutical profession and entertained by Bell and Redwood, Liebig visited the Pharmaceutical Society and its laboratories. Langdon Down saw Liebig as a possible mentor and he probably met him during his time at the Pharmaceutical Society. Alternatively, Redwood may have taken Langdon Down along to the house of his father-in-law, a Mr Morson, in Southampton Row, where Liebig was also a frequent visitor.

In his letter he wrote: 'in the event of nothing turning up I should be very well fitted for the chemist's counter, possessing for my move, I hope, a fund of information which no bankruptcy can take away'[1]. He asked Philip Crellin for advice about other prospects of salaried positions, such as that of an assistant at Crystal Palace. Here was a young man who was desperate to be independent and strike out on his own, but the prospect of being able to follow his first choice of career appeared to be remote.

As circumstances evolved, his problem was solved by his sister Sarah and her husband Philip Crellin. They offered him board and lodging in London to begin his medical studies in the autumn. His mother helped as well. She was anxious about the fact that Philip and Sarah Crellin were providing him with all his meals and fires in his room and, with some difficulty, persuaded them to accept a weekly payment from her of five shillings, approximately £15 in today's terms.

The fees at the London Hospital, where he ultimately began his studies, were 85 guineas, somewhat higher than at the Middlesex. The fee for attendance at the formal lectures and for clinical tuition was 94 guineas. In addition there was a three guinea registration fee. He had this saved. The Crellins, who took him as a non-paying guest, had no children of their own, then or later. Their house was his base throughout the entire period of his studies and his mother considered him to be very fortunate to have such a kind sister and brother-in-law who would allow of this arrangement[2].

The medical school lectures included courses in anatomy, physiology, chemistry, medicine, surgery, midwifery, materia medica, ophthalmic surgery, botany, forensic medicine, comparative anatomy, practical chemistry and practical histology. In addition students acted as dressers in the surgical department of the hospital and as clinical clerks in the medical department. It was their duty to record the progress of patients and report on any changes. They had to present their findings in detail to members of the visiting staff and discuss them at the bedside. Medicine was entirely a clinical science. The X-ray machine had not yet been invented and laboratory investigations were extremely limited. Langdon Down was assigned to Dr Little. Little later thought so highly of him as a student that he presented him with a copy of his new textbook *The Nature and Treatment of Deformities of the Human Frame*. He inscribed it 'JH Langdon Down, esq., as a mark of esteem and respect for his ability and attainments by his teacher WJ Little'[3].

The emphasis was on detailed history taking, thorough inspection of the patient, palpation of all organs possible, including their

LECTURES

ON

DEFORMITIES OF THE HUMAN FRAME.

Dr WJ Little, a senior physician at the London Hospital, presented Langdon Down with an inscribed copy of his famous textbook. The inscription reads: 'JH Langdon Down Esq., as a mark of esteem and respect for his ability and attainments by his teacher WJ Little'.

delineation by finger percussion and, finally, the use of the stethoscope. This had only recently become a standard part of the doctor's equipment, but John Langdon Down became competent in its use for chest infections. In the London Hospital he had learned cardiology from Dr Herbert Davies whose lecture notes covered diseases of the heart valves, aneurysms and vegetations. There was, as yet, no great interest in the detailed diagnosis of congenital heart disease. No treatments were available and so definitive diagnosis would only have been academic. In dealing with a patient who had circulatory problems, he simply described the circulation as weak. It was to be another 20 years before definitive signs of specific types of congenital heart disease became defined. Just as he had been an outstanding student at the Royal Pharmaceutical Society, he quickly proved himself once more at the London Hospital. The list of his successes marked him as a brilliant student.

He first entered the London Hospital under the auspices of the Worshipful Society of Apothecaries, whose Licentiate he was to take three years later. The Licentiate, which he took concurrently with the membership of the Royal College of Surgeons, would have entitled him to be registered and practise medicine as a general practitioner (GP). In June 1854 he matriculated in parallel in the University of London, having perhaps perceived that a university degree might enable him to reach a higher level of acceptance in the medical profession. In the university matriculation examination he was awarded a special prize in chemistry. The University of London required candidates to sit two examinations. In the first of these he won an exhibition and a gold medal in materia medica and an exhibition and a gold medal in chemistry, in addition to passing the examination in botany with honours. These two exhibitions were worth £50 each for two years, enough to cover his living expenses. The first professional examination he took was on 7 April 1856 when the court of examiners of the Royal College of Surgeons passed John Langdon Haydon Down, candidate number 5100.

There was, however, an element of irregularity in the Royal College's assent to Langdon Down's presenting himself for the examination, as his formal professional training had been of three years duration and not four, as required[4]. Presumably the Royal College took into account his certificate of having been an indentured apprentice to his father. His father had in fact died on 5 August, 1853, the year before Langdon Down's period of apprenticeship as an apothecary was to have been completed. He was clearly a young man of great promise and both the Royal College and the Worshipful Society of Apothecaries' appear to have made concessions to allow him to take the qualifying examinations, although technically not yet qualified to do so.

The format of the examination has changed over the years. The qualifying examination in medicine at the present time requires an assessment of clinical skills in addition to theoretical knowledge but, in 1856, the qualifying examination of the Royal College of Surgeons took the form of an oral assessment. A court of examiners, headed by the President and Vice-president met each week to examine prospective candidates. Langdon Down was examined by William Lawrence, Surgeon Extraordinary to the Queen and Professor of Anatomy and Surgery in the College; Benjamin Travers, Surgeon in Ordinary to the Queen, and Edward Stanley, Surgeon to St Bartholomew's Hospital. He satisfied the examiners, paid his fees and now had a registrable medical qualification.

He presented for the Licentiate of the Worshipful Society of Apothecaries on 13 November, 1856. This examination, like that for the primary qualification for the Royal College of Surgeons, was entirely theoretical. A prospective candidate was required to produce a testimonial of having served an apprenticeship of not less than five years to an apothecary. The certifying apothecary must have satisfied the requirements of the 1815 Act or else to have received a certificate of qualification from the Court of Examiners of the Society. Candidates had to be 21 years of age, verified, if possible, by a baptismal certificate, be of good moral conduct, and to have pursued a course of medical study in conformity with the regulations of the Court. The testimonial of moral character should, if possible, be from the gentleman to whom the candidate had been apprenticed. In Langdon Down's case, his father being dead, the testimonial of moral character was signed by his brother-in-law, Phillip Crellin.

The early 1800s was a time of flux and change in the relationship between pharmacists and physicians. The Worshipful Society of Apothecaries, founded in 1617, conducted examinations which included a strong element of assessment of competence in dispensing drugs. In practice an apothecary was a GP who also dispensed the drugs which he prescribed. Even in this century dispensing practices have continued to operate, especially in rural areas where GPs, who do not have access to pharmacy service, dispense their own drugs. The Apothecaries Act of 1815[5] allowed an apothecary to prescribe treatment as well as to dispense drugs and apothecaries were eligible to act as medical practitioners.

The 1815 Act also required the Society to exercise quality control, by visiting apothecaries' shops and examining the purity of medicaments. From 1 August, 1815 it was illegal to practise as an apothecary in any part of England or Wales without having a certificate from the Society. The Society was required to publish a list of those qualified each year, and nobody was allowed to qualify as an apothecary without passing an examination conducted by the Society's Court of Examiners. The examiners had to ascertain the candidates' skill and abilities in the science and practice of medicine and their fitness and qualification to practise as an apothecary.

There was however a 'grandfather' clause which allowed for apothecaries who were in practice before 1815 to continue to claim apothecaries' fees. It was not necessary for them to register with the Worshipful Society; they could simply declare themselves to be apothecaries de facto and the issue only became important if they sued for their fees through the courts. In this instance the apothecary had to prove in court that he had been in practice before the 1815 Act. However, if he avoided the courts, his self-declared occupation of apothecary would not be challenged. Joseph Almond Down may have declared himself to be an apothecary solely for the purpose of signing an indenture certificate for his son. The indenture is dated January 1st 1849 (see Appendix 1).

Although the formal instruction required was three winter sessions of six months each and two summer sessions of three months each, totalling 24 months, Langdon Down's certificate refers to a 15 month period of attendance. Under practical chemistry he is noted as being excused by the Court, presumably as a result of his having taken the examination of the Royal Pharmaceutical Society and the preliminary examination of the London University examination in medicine.

The content of the examination was orientated towards the multiple skills required of an apothecary. He was expected to translate portions of both the first four books of *Celsus de Medicina* and the first 23 chapters of Gregory's *Conspectus Medicinae Theoreticae*, physicians' prescriptions, and the *Pharmacopoeia Londinensis*. The examination covered chemistry, practical chemistry, materia medica and therapeutics, botany, anatomy, physiology and the principles and practice of medicine, including midwifery and the diseases of children. Once again the examination was entirely theoretical, apart from the emphasis on the writing of prescriptions. Langdon Down had not fully completed the period of training laid down by either of the qualifying bodies. In the examination setting, however, he would clearly have impressed both Courts with the wealth of his knowledge; technical deficiencies in his certificates were therefore overlooked.

Langdon Down was now entitled to practise medicine. As a London Hospital student he was a bright star in the academic firmament. He was awarded the three hospital gold medals, one in each of the major examination subjects – medicine, surgery and obstetrics. In addition he was awarded the gold medal for the best clinical student of his year. He had studied long and hard and emerged as a brilliant student and a keen observer. As soon as he had passed the examinations for the Membership of the Royal College of Surgeons and the licence of the Worshipful Society of Apothecaries in 1856, he was headhunted and appointed obstetric resident or accoucheur in the London Hospital. This appointment was for six months but he made such an impact that he was re-appointed three times, until September 1858. The standing orders of the hospital were suspended in order to allow this. The appointment was unpaid but he was entitled to free board and lodging and so to a degree was now independent.

His work as resident accoucheur was arduous. He was required to live in the hospital, not to absent himself by day or night without the permission of his House Governor and only then if he had left the name of a qualified and acceptable substitute. He was to visit every inpatient daily and to summon the Obstetric Physician for all emergencies. He was to attend all urgent or dangerous maternity cases when summoned by the attending medical student and to attend to all cases where the allocated attending student was not available. In addition, it was his duty to allocate students to the booked cases and keep records of the outcome. Discipline among the students was difficult to maintain and he undoubtedly had to take responsibility for cases assigned to medical students who could not be found at the appointed hour. The resident accoucheur was also to hold a vaccination clinic each Monday morning. In addition he was expected to give an example of circumspection and propriety and to attend Divine Worship regularly in the hospital chapel[6].

Langdon Down was under the direction of Dr Francis Ramsbotham, the first official obstetric teacher in the hospital. Francis Ramsbotham's textbook on the principles of obstetric

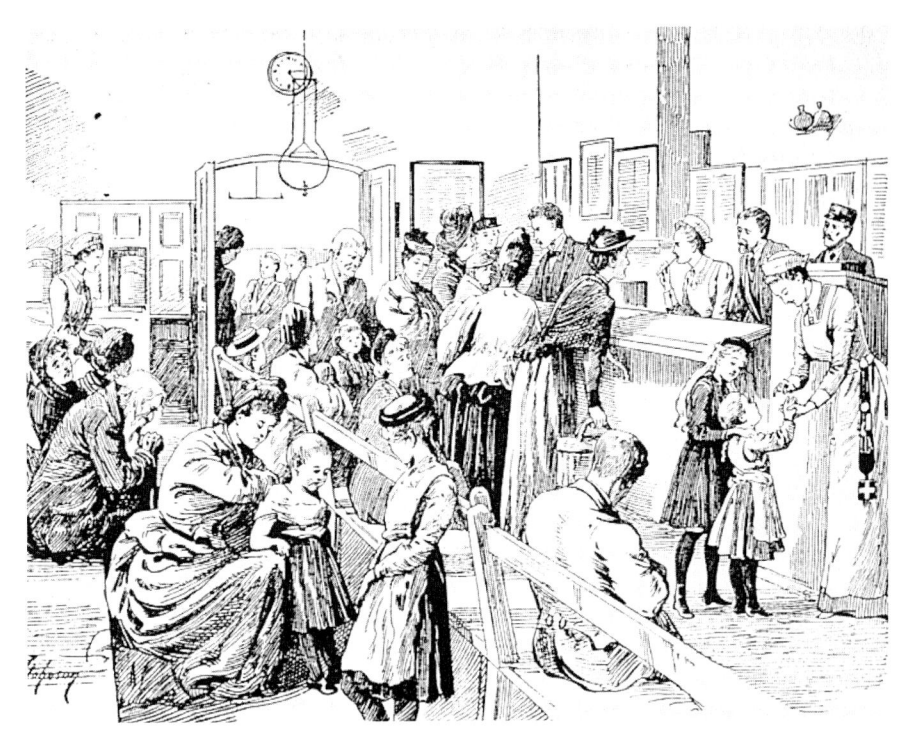

The outpatient department at the London Hospital. The hospital served the poor of the East End. From The Illustrated London News, *1886.*

medicine and surgery reached its fourth edition in 1855[7]. There was no separate obstetric inpatient unit and obstetric patients were accommodated on the medical and surgical wards. The scale of the hospital activity can be judged from the tables published by Ramsbotham in his textbook covering the years 1820 to 1827 when, on average, 2600 births were handled each year on the extern service. The statistics for the intern service for 1858–63 showed 390 patients being admitted each year.

Childbirth was hazardous and 15 mothers died in one year, 10 from peritonitis – a devastating maternal mortality of 3.8%. Langdon Down was learning the hard way. Ramsbotham's book showed the range of his knowledge and his experience; there was in particular a long appendix on the resuscitation of infants with suspended animation, or delayed spontaneous breathing and on congenital malformations[7]. Langdon Down profited greatly from this experience and, when he later came to discuss the causation of idiocy, he referred, with respect and appreciation, to Ramsbotham's training[8]. Langdon Down was also assistant lecturer in comparative anatomy during this period and in 1856 he took on, in addition, the role of medical tutor. *The Medical Directory* for these years does not list these additional appointments under the London Hospital entry

A signed copy of Nature's Balance, *Langdon Down's prize essay, given to Mary Crellin 'with the best wishes of the author'. They married in 1860.*

and the titles may have been informal, but they generated some small income. The students having difficulty with their examinations frequently sought and paid for special tutorials and this was no doubt very welcome.

In the house of his sister, Sarah and her husband Philip Crellin, Philip's sister, Mary, was a frequent visitor. She was an able and cultured woman, fluent in French and a talented pianist. She was warm-hearted, lively and witty and in time showed herself to be an exceptionally capable administrator. The relationship between her and John advanced from friendship to affection and ultimately to thoughts of marriage. They were both religious people and, before they were on first name terms, he gave her a signed copy of his prize essay on 'The Wisdom of God', which she treasured all her life. It is still in the hands of the family. She read it many times and underlined the salient points in pencil.

Marriage, which they ultimately came to discuss, was at the time out of the question. Even if his career were to advance to an ultimate appointment to the staff of the London Hospital, he would still have to face years of impecunious struggle. Voluntary hospital appointments were unpaid and private practice would take time to develop. Substantial funding was needed if they were to marry unless he had the good fortune to obtain a salaried post, of which there were very few. A career in medicine could not easily be matched with the requirements of a home and family and there was no shortcut to success. A man might expect to take between five and seven years to establish a viable consulting practice and these years of struggle and striving would be spent in relative poverty, depending on the low cash flow of tutorial work and occasional locum fees and consultations.

With his certificate of qualification as an apothecary it was open to Langdon Down to become a GP, renting premises for a surgery and hoping and waiting for patients to register. His sights, were, however, set on higher things and, while doing duty as obstetric resident, he continued as a student until he took the MB degree of examination of London University, where he again distinguished himself. He was awarded an honours degree and placed second overall in the University examination. He was to move quickly to higher qualifications and within a year of his taking up his next post in the Earlswood Asylum for Idiots, he passed the MD examination of the University of London. University regulations at that time did not require a candidate to submit either a thesis or a dissertation, although these were later required. There is no record of him presenting a thesis and he presumably took the degree by examination. He passed the Membership examination of the Royal College of Physicians in the same year. The usual time lag between passing the MB examination and succeeding in the membership examination is ordinarily about three years and his accelerated progress was clearly a sign of exceptional ability.

References

1 Letter to Philip Crellin, May 2nd, 1849. Unpublished correspondence, courtesy of Lord Christopher Brain.
2 Letter from Sarah Crellin, undated, probably November 1896. Unpublished correspondence, courtesy of Lord Christopher Brain.

3   Brain R. The Neurological Tradition of the London Hospital. *London Hospital Gazette* 1959; 62(suppl); **62**: iii–xv.
4   Royal College of Surgeons Calendar. Examination Regulations. *Medical Directory*, 1855.
5   Act for better regulating the practice of apothecaries, 1815.
6   London Hospital Regulations, 1856.
7   Ramsbotham J. *The Practice of Midwifery*. Churchill, 1855.
8   Down JLD. *The Obstetrical Aspects of Idiocy in Mental Affections of Childhood and Youth*. Churchill, 1887.

── Chapter 5 ──

The Royal Earlswood Asylum for Idiots

In 1858 his whole life and career irrevocably changed. During a family summer break, Miss Jolly, a friend of his sister, mentioned that her father and brother – who were subscribers to the Royal Earlswood Asylum for Idiots in Redhill, Surrey – had let her know that the Asylum was to look for a new Medical Superintendent. Langdon Down moved quickly to canvass support for his candidacy for this post. This was a salaried appointment and had the additional attraction that married quarters were provided. The only specific qualifications required were either a medical degree from a British university or the double qualification of membership of the Royal College of Surgeons conjoined with the Licentiate of the Worshipful Society of Apothecaries. Langdon Down had all of these.

The Earlswood Asylum for Idiots was the brainchild of the Reverend Dr Andrew Reed, prompted by Mrs Rowland Plumbe, one of his parishioners. Dr Reed had entered the ministry of the Congregational Church in 1811 and, in 1831, had become minister of the highly successful Wycliffe Chapel. He was a well-known philanthropist and had himself seen wretched instances of the handicapped being chained like villains or maniacs in the common pound, or in the lock-up house on the village green. 'I think', he wrote, 'from the observations I have made that an Asylum is greatly needed for indigent idiots. Enquiry must be made and, if needed, action must follow. In all the land' he said, 'with all its hospitals and charities there is no asylum for the poor idiot at all'[1]. He approached the problem with missionary zeal. His philosophy about those affected was: 'some are better, some worse, this is the maximum of incapacity: but the Divine image is stamped on all'.

He visited Paris, Germany and Switzerland and invited Johann Guggenbuhl to come from Abendberg to give his advice. His associate in the endeavour, Sir John Forbes, entered into a conditional agreement with Guggenbuhl that one of his Lutheran Sisters of Charity would come to England to assist in the operation of a proposed new home in Highgate, but it would appear that the Sister never came. Dr Reed opened correspondence with medical men in different foreign cities who had made the management of learning disability their specialty.

Andrew Reed was a great campaigner and realized that the project would need support from the leaders of society. At a meeting in the Kings Head Tavern on 20 July, 1847, it was agreed that the care of idiots should be distinguished from the care of the insane. Whatever accommodation was available at that time for the handicapped was confined to lunatic asylums. He then moved into the corridors of political power and mustered a team of subscribers of such eminence that the list reads like a page from *Debrett's Peerage* – two Dukes, two Marquises, seven Earls and seven Lords, together with the Viscount Ebrington and, on the clerical side, the Archbishop of Canterbury supported by five Bishops. At various times other peers, including Lord Ashby and Baron Rothschild, held office on the Board of Governors. In total there were ultimately 10,000 subscribers[2].

These important contacts in due course gave Langdon Down a high clinical and social profile. The wealthy subscribers to the Asylum came to know him and, when he later set up his private institution and practice, wealthy families knew they could turn to him for help and did. He had a captive audience of 10,000 whom he could address; they were marshalled by rich and famous leaders of society who, in turn, attracted the support of the upwardly mobile middle classes. His annual reports were sent to all subscribers and they all came to know the stature of the man.

At the meeting to launch the project, the Chair was taken by Sir George Carroll, the Lord Mayor of London and an address prepared by Dr Reed was read by Mr Charles Gilpin MP. Dr Reed was himself the first subscriber, the second being the 'widowed mother of an idiot child, who in gratitude contributed her ten guineas'. Following the opening public meeting on 17 October, 1847 in the London Tavern, a house was purchased in Highgate and opened in March of the following year. In the first report Dr Reed set out his philosophy in the management of patients, the main priority being education[1]. The first principle he laid down was that there was, in every instance, a mind that in itself was perfect, but that it had imperfect and defective expression or imperfect or defective organization. The hope was that by training the eye, ear, mouth, muscles and limbs, patients might advance. It was hoped that they might also be trained to moral and spiritual exercises. This would, of course, require great patience and it was wrong to think that everything could be accomplished in weeks or even months.

There had to be a patience of labour and energy of benevolence which knew no weariness and which refused to be discouraged. The first experiences were a challenge even to the most resolute and they would not be forgotten at the time by any who experienced them. Patients were clamorous and rebellious, some sullen and perverse, some unconscious and inert and some screaming at the top of their voices, or making constant involuntary noises from nervous irritation. Some were petrified at scorn and ill treatment and hid themselves in corners away from men, as from an enemy. Windows were smashed, wainscotting broken and a spirit of mischief and disobedience prevailed. It seemed as though nothing except prison accommodation would meet the needs of such a group. Many who saw these scenes of disorder retired in disgust or despair. With kindly management and order, obedience to authority and cheerful occupation gradually emerged. This was all secured without the aid of correction or coercion. The principle which ruled the institution was Love and Charity – Divine Charity[1].

The second matter for concern was the permanent care of the 'idiot'. There was a need for long-term services for the most severely affected. It had to be accepted that there were cases which would allow of little improvement and, even if improvement came, the sufferers were disqualified from fulfilling the duties of life and were unable to resist the trials and temptations of a bustling and selfish world. He addressed rhetorical questions: 'Are they to be abandoned because they inspire little hope and need the most care? Is it nothing to make them safe? To redeem them from misery and scorn? To find them a home? To provide them with suitable occupation and to save them from vacancy and fatuity?'[1].

Initially admission was confined to the middle classes, neither paying patients or pauper cases being admitted. Paying patients came to be admitted later which contributed to the financial stability of Earlswood. In the unpublished account of Earlswood by Christopher Crayon in 1887 a passage indicates that the wealthy were seen as making a positive contribution. Christopher Crayon was the pseudonym of the author Ewing Ritchie. He wrote:

> The wealthy and the noble are as likely to have idiotic children as any other class of the community... No wonder that the rich idiots in Earlswood have been numerous. They pay, of course, handsomely; no charitable funds are appropriated to them and they are handsomely treated... At one time they came almost exclusively to Earlswood and acted not a little to keep such an enormous establishment, conducted necessarily on such an expensive scale, in funds. Other rival establishments have now come in to the field to cater for the wealthy classes; but some such are at Earlswood still[3].

Dr Reed's influence was everywhere. He busied himself with the selection of masters, nurses and servants and in the organization of contracts for supplies, the preparation of a gymnasium and the laying out of garden allotments. His belief was that one in three affected children could be greatly restored and he hoped that his good work 'would make them the merriest family in green England'[1]. The pressure of numbers made it necessary to move the younger inmates to Essex Hall in Colchester. The Queen sent for Dr Reed and made the Prince of Wales a life patron. An address, presented by Alderman Abbiss to the Corporation of London, led to a contribution of 200 guineas, (£120,000 today) and this example was followed by many other public bodies. In 1852 Judge Talfourd relinquished a site in Redhill for the erection of a new institution. The foundation stone was laid by the Prince Consort in June in the same year. By 1855 a building large enough for 500 residents had been erected. It was opened by the Prince Consort and blessed by Samuel Wilberforce, the Bishop of Oxford. It had cost £30,000 to build.

A number of medical men of great eminence assisted Dr Reed with advice. The famous John Conolly – who had abolished all forms of personal restraint in the lunatic asylum at Hanwell, of which he was Superintendent – was Andrew Reed's principal advisor. He was one of a group of public-spirited Dissenters recruited by Dr Reed for this huge project. He was, in time, to influence John Langdon Down in his thinking. Conolly's ideas are well-illustrated in the letter he wrote on 17 October, 1860 to Dr Brown, the Commissioner in Lunacy for Scotland, when he was trying to influence him in establishing an Earlswood style institution in Scotland. He wrote:

> The spectacle of 300 children there assembled – each child rescued from solitude and neglect, from misery, from semi-starvation, from mockery and persecution – is one that does honour to humanity. The cleanliness, the order, the comfort of all the apartments; the extensive grounds and pleasant gardens in which so many groups of children are generally seen, some at play, some at work, and all pleased to see the visitors, whom they approach with confidence and trust, and even with affection; the schools in which they are variously educated, and with never ceasing patience and

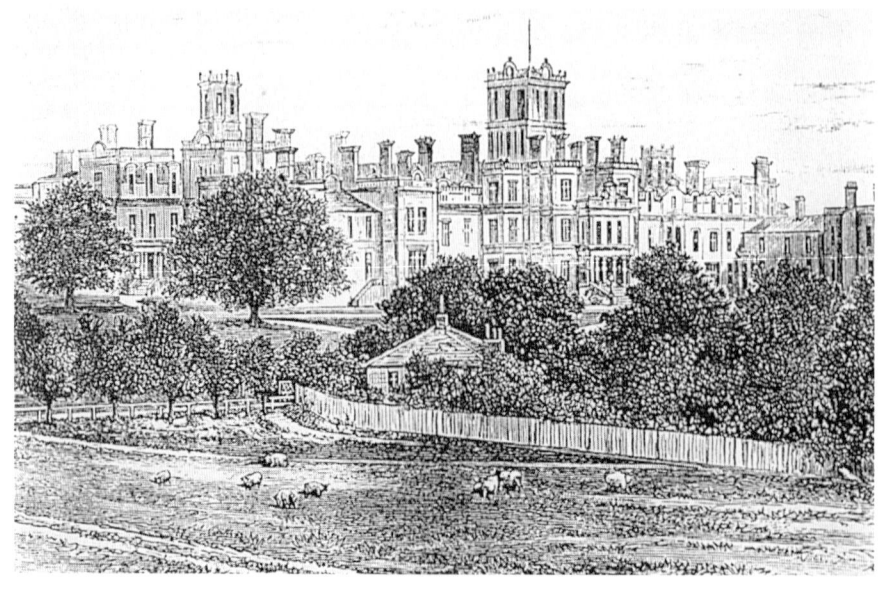

The Royal Earlswood Asylum for Idiots, Redhill, Surrey, in 1880.

kindness; the workshops in which they are taught many useful occupations; the abundant and good food provided for them; the various amusements and recreations; the large hall in which they meet on different occasions, and in which their voices are so often to be heard united in simple prayer, or thanks and devotional song; all these things combine to give a distinct character to the establishment, as one where goodness and mercy prevailed, and to form a scene most impressive upon all who take an interest in the poor creatures, who are the least finished among the works of the Creator of all things[4].

The religious emphasis was always maintained and the residents were taken to Sunday worship. On account of the residents' learning difficulties, religious instruction was to be of the simplest character; it was decided that they should learn the Lord's Prayer, the Ten Commandments and the Apostles' Creed. There were also formal morning and evening prayers in line with the spirit of the institution. Dr Reed emphasized the importance of high quality staff; the raising of the standard of recruitment had always been a priority with John Conolly and this had been one of his basic reforms in Hanwell. They were to be entrusted with the happiness of their patients by day and night. They should control the violent without anger, soothe the irritable without weak and foolish concessions, cheer and comfort the depressed, guard the imbecile and impulsive and direct all.

The second medical advisor was WJ Little. He had entered on his medical career as an apprentice to an apothecary in East London and later studied at the London Hospital. He suffered from club foot, possibly following poliomyelitis. During a spell in Germany, he persuaded the famous surgeon, Stromeyer to carry out a tendon lengthening operation so that he could put his heel to the ground. The results were very satisfactory and he went on to learn the surgical technique himself and to become an expert on the surgical correction of deformities.

His name is commemorated in the description of the form of cerebral palsy which affects the legs more than the arms, which he described, now called Little's disease[5]. In this noteworthy paper he discussed the effect of difficult labour, premature birth, asphyxia and other complicating factors of delivery on the mental and physical condition of the infant, especially in relation to deformities. Little canvassed actively in support of Langdon Down's appointment and not only wrote a testimonial on his behalf but also approached Sir John Forbes, the third of the eminent medical men associated with the institution as well as approaching Dr Reed directly.

Sir John Forbes was Physician in Ordinary to the Royal Household. He was also a Fellow of the Royal College of Physicians and the Royal Society, a prolific author and editor of two medical journals. In the 1820s and 1830s he wrote books on the use of the stethoscope, with which the medical profession was only then becoming familiar. He was also the editor of a medical encyclopedia. He was a man of influence and stature in the corridors of power and, as a medical man, was held in high regard by society at large. His influence in Earlswood was very important; he and Conolly were the elder statesmen who were called upon to solve medical problems in the administration of the Asylum. Their association with the Institution gave it public credibility and contributed to its acceptance.

John Conolly had visited the Bicêtre Hospital in Paris to see Edouard Séguin and study his techniques. He had reported in the *British and Foreign Medical Gazette* on what he had seen. In the same journal in 1847 an anonymous review of Séguin's book on the Moral Treatment was published, possibly penned and certainly read by him[6]. In spite of the high ideals and great expectations of its founders, the Earlswood Asylum for Idiots got off to a bad start, possibly because its founders had so much to do and tried to do it too quickly. The Commissioners in Lunacy were alarmed by what they saw.

Earlswood's Previous Problems

The starry-eyed enthusiasm of its founders had led to the opening of Earlswood before everything had been fully prepared. The Commissioners in Lunacy, who had statutory responsibility for regular inspection of the Asylum, wrote in 1856 that there were 146 patients[7]. They all appeared to be in reasonable health and the girls were generally clean and well-clothed but some of the boys were dirty, untidy and offensive in their persons and dress. The girls' rooms were in fair condition but the boys' wards and the offices, except for the kitchen, were in a very unsatisfactory state. In many rooms the floors were sanded and very dirty. The walls were stained and the grates uncleaned. There was a dangerous practice of lighting fires without the protection of a fender. The dining hall, which had been used during the summer, could not be used in winter because there was no heating.

The back yards were wet, muddy and almost impassable. The washhouse was in a very dirty and offensive condition. 'The bedding was much stained and some was rotten[7]'. There was an unsatisfactory practice of simply putting a clean coverlet over the mattress during the day, conveying a false impression of cleanliness. The atmosphere in one of the dormitories was very offensive and in several of the bedrooms washstands had been installed as the lavatories were not working. The water supply was unsatisfactory as the water was brown, turbid and quite unsuited for drinking purposes.

Four years after it opened, the boys' playground was still unfit for use and paths through the ground were so soft that they could rarely be used in the winter months. In consequence of the bad materials of which the paths were made the patients, in particular the girls, were very much confined to the house during the winter. The Commissioners recommended that all residents be provided with strong and suitable shoes and that a shoe room be provided so that patients could change their shoes on returning from outdoors. They were particularly scathing about the statutory records as they found that these were entirely neglected. No entry whatever had been made in the medical visitation book and no particulars of medical treatment had been recorded. The Commissioners drew the attention of the Medical Superintendent to the provision of the Act of Parliament under which the Institution operated. This set out that his neglect to maintain the records had made him liable to very heavy financial penalties, apart from the issue of neglecting a most obvious and important duty.

The Commissioners recommended that steps be taken immediately to improve the management and internal condition of the Institution which did not, in their opinion, properly carry out the benevolent intentions of the founders and subscribers. The Commissioners recommended that a sub-committee of the Governors be set up with full power to issue whatever directions were necessary in order to bring the establishment into full and efficient operation. One year later no sub-committee had been appointed and, although some minor improvements had been made, the condition of the Asylum was very much as before.

The Commissioners were concerned that the great benefit which would result from employing the patients in industrial pursuits, which had been repeatedly suggested, had not advanced. They recommended once more that the residents be employed in household work, the laundry, the garden and various trades and that they should be taught to wash and dress themselves, to keep themselves clean and neat and, by adhering to these measures, also diminish the expense of running the Asylum. Although the Asylum had its own bakery, bread was being brought in from outside. Meat was being sent in open baskets from Kensington and, because of the great distance involved, it was sometimes unfit for consumption during the hot weather.

The problem of wet and dirty beds was referred to repeatedly and in 1858 the Commissioners were concerned that no effort was being made to correct these faulty habits. They took the view that no case of incontinence was hopeless and that the night staff should be directed to educate the pupils to attend the calls of nature and that the number of night attendants should be increased so that all incontinent pupils should be directly supervised. Worse was to follow but the House Committee endeavoured to effect some improvements[8]. They directed that no fires be lit in any room without a fender and that sand be scattered on the dining room floor to prevent grease spots. They curtained the dining room and glazed the openings into the foyer. They directed that the bedding for the dirty cases be reconsidered and expressed regret that there should have been any neglect of the statutory records. The attention of the Medical Superintendent was called to this by special resolution. Finances were a problem and the annual payment for paying cases was reviewed. On full consideration it was left to stand at £100 (£6,000 in current terms).

There was clearly concern about the manner in which the Medical Superintendent conducted his affairs. In June 1857 he was directed to keep himself free from all official engagements and to devote all his time to the service of the Board, with office hours from 9.30 am to 5 pm except when, in the opinion of the Board, the pressure of business required that he should attend for longer hours. The Superintendent should give specific directions concerning the potential of individual patients so that, in the school or in any particular occupation, the schoolmaster or the attendant should be aware of the physical powers of the patient. He was to keep a daily journal and a casebook, which should contain as full a history as could be set out in each case, together with an indication of the probable cause of the existing mental or bodily infirmity. The progress of each case should, from time to time, be recorded in the same book. Under the 1845 Act 'For the Regulation of Care and Treatment of Lunatics' the Medical Superintendent was liable to a fine of £10 for any neglect in keeping the casebook according to the form directed by the Commissioners. A special enquiry was also initiated into a practice which the medical superintendent had allowed to develop, of permitting attendants on night duty to sleep in a separate room from the patients. This had been done without the consent of the Committee. In October 1857 Dr Conolly and Sir John Forbes set out to enquire into the negative report of the Commissioners in Lunacy in the hope that all relevant points could be gone into, explained and refuted.

An even greater scandal emerged in 1858. A patient called Matilda J was admitted with a history of severe diarrhoea[9]. Her feet were noted to be discoloured and were wrapped in cotton wool. They remained bandaged and were not looked at again for five days when an offensive smell prompted the removal of the dressings. Five of her toes had become gangrenous and had sloughed off and it appeared that the other five toes would also soon be lost. Dr Maxwell's response to a House Committee enquiry was that he had been unwell over the period in question and that he had relied on the nursing staff to inform him if there had been a change in the patient's condition, but had not himself visited her over the five-day period. He offered his resignation but asked that it should be postponed until the case of Matilda J had been finally resolved. Her parents had communicated the facts to the Commissioners in Lunacy but he did not wish to have it appear that his resignation had been forced.

Sir John Forbes and Dr Conolly were deputed to investigate the matter and they concluded that there had been no medical negligence. The Commissioners in Lunacy investigated the matter further and their report was as follows:

> We have made an enquiry into the case of a little girl, Matilda J. who lost the toes of both feet from mortification in the month of January last. The attention of the Commissioners was drawn to this case by the child's mother, but the investigation was conducted by the Committee, whom she had also addressed on the subject. The final result of the enquiry has not been communicated to us. As far as we can judge the greatest blame attaches to the nurse who was in charge of the case.
>
> It appears that the child being of feeble constitution orders had been given by Dr Maxwell to the head nurse that her feet should be rubbed and kept warm. On January 25th the head nurse looked at Jenner's feet and found them dark coloured, without any sores. She then rubbed them, applied resin ointment and cotton wool and put on stockings. From this time up to the 29th no further examination of the feet seems to have been made, but the attention of the under-nurse being attracted by an offensive odour proceeding from the child's feet, the dressings were removed and the toes were found to be in a state of mortification.
>
> Dr Maxwell informs us that during the period from the 15th to the 28th he was confined to bed and his duties were performed by Dr Martin of Reigate. We are surprised to find that in spite of these circumstances the head nurse Huxley is still employed in the Institution. We learn from Dr Maxwell that he has tendered his resignation and will leave the Hospital in the month of September. We therefore take this opportunity of urging upon the Committee the great importance of attaching such a salary to the office of Superintendent as may secure the services of a thoroughly efficient and competent officer. In our opinion Dr Maxwell never had sufficient power delegated to him and we think it is essential to the wellbeing of this Institution that his successor should have full control, not only over the other officers and servants, but also in the general management of the establishment. The Medical superintendent should publish a report annually upon the general condition of the hospital[10].

Dr Maxwell tendered his resignation in June, to take effect in September. The Committee agreed that, by way of compensation to the family, the patient should be maintained free of charge for five years. This new development came at a time when the Asylum had attracted adverse publicity in the newspapers and there was some discussion on suing the *Telegraph*, which had published an adverse commentary on the report of the Commissioners in Lunacy. Dr Conolly lamented the fact that the Institution, which had been intended to be a model to be looked up to from all quarters, had certainly got into bad repute. The Commissioners had made various suggestions and these should be acted on. A sub-committee consisting of Drs Little and Conolly and Sir John Forbes was set up to fill the vacant office of Medical Superintendent. The salary for the post should be £400 per annum (£24,000 today). Any lower salary would not be sufficient to attract a gentleman of merit and worth.

When the news of the impending appointment of a Superintendent filtered out through the subscribers, Langdon Down went to see Dr Little of the London Hospital. Little strongly advised him to apply. Dr Little had already suggested to Dr Reed that Langdon Down would be the right man for the job. In his testimonial he said:

> I have been acquainted with Mr Langdon Down over several years and have been much gratified by the assiduity, intelligence and general ability manifested by him in the various capacities in which he has been occupied at the hospital (The London Hospital). He is deeply versed in the higher branches of professional and scientific knowledge, he has much experience in both medical and surgical diseases, he has acquired the regard and confidence of the Authorities of the Hospital and is in my opinion peculiarly qualified for the post of Medical Superintendent to the Idiots Asylum at Earlswood[11].

He wrote a personal note to Sir John Forbes drawing attention to his previous recommendation to Dr Reed that Langdon Down would be a very reliable person for Earlswood 'You will find him an uncommonly well-informed man[11]'.

Francis Ramsbotham, the head of the Obstetric Department in which Langdon Down had worked for two years, also wrote to Sir John: 'I would very much like to interest you in favour of my friend Mr Down who is a candidate for the office of Medical Superintendent. He is MB University of London and holds two exhibitions from it. He has for two years been my assistant at the London Hospital and is altogether one of the cleverest fellows I know. He ran away with all our prizes as a student. If you elect him I am sure you will congratulate yourselves on having done so[11]'. An even more fulsome recommendation came from Dr Clark; he wrote:

> I am conscious of the responsibility assumed in speaking of the fitness of anyone for such an office; I know that the holder of it

must possess a rare combination of natural and acquired qualifications; that he must be impressed with a high and correct idea of his functions, that his whole heart must be in his work... Mr Down's collegiate career was one of unvarying and unexampled success. At university examinations he gained the highest honours in several departments. His diligence, humanity and skill in the hospital wards elicited the approbation of the Authorities. He only ceased to be a pupil when he was made a teacher and chosen for a resident appointment in the hospital which familiarized him with the working of one of the best conducted institutions in the Kingdom... If he were appointed Superintendent to the Asylum he would perform duties of the office with benefit and satisfaction to all concerned; and that he would so use his opportunities for the investigation of truth and bring so many kinds of knowledge to bear upon it that he would scarcely fail to extend the reputation of the Asylum and to prove otherwise subservient the good of mankind and the Glory of God[11].

Langdon Down also had the support of the Reverend Canon Champneys. The letter of clerical support set out that he had been the means of conferring the greatest benefits upon multitudes of poor women and children in the neighbourhood of the London Hospital. He was well known to the clergy, by name, for his great kindness to the poor, whom he visited day and night in their wretched homes over a period of two years. He was considered to be a man of great talent and moral worth and the London Hospital would sustain a heavy loss if he were appointed to Earlswood. These and several other testimonials are lodged in the London Metropolitan Records Office[11].

Coincidentally a vacancy had arisen at the same time in the London Hospital, for an assistant physician. Langdon Down, having called on various governors, as was customary, to solicit their support found that they had already committed themselves to Dr Hughlings Jackson. He wrote withdrawing his application to the London Hospital in the light of the various governors' prior commitment. Within a year it had been decided to appoint an additional assistant physician and, on this occasion, Langdon Down was to be the successful candidate.

References

1 Surrey Record Office. SRO;392/1/2/1. First annual report.
2 Surrey Record Office. SRO;392/1/2/1. List of subscribers.
3 Crayon C. *All About Earlswood*. Earlswood Museum, Surrey.
4 Clark J. *A Memoir of John Conolly*. London: John Murray, 1869.
5 Little WJ. On the influences of abnormal parturition. *Obst Trans* 1862; **3**: 293–346.

6 Séguin E. *The Moral Treatment, Hygiene and Education of Idiots, Review.*
7 Surrey Record Office. SRO;392/10/1/1. Visitor's report, 1856.
8 Surrey Record Office. SRO;392/2/2/2. Annual Reports. Twelfth Report of the Commissioners in Lunacy, 1858.
9 Surrey Record Office. SRO;392/3/1/3. Annual Reports, 1858.
10 Surrey Record Office. SRO;392/10/1/1. Report of Visiting Medical Officers.
11 London Metropolitan Records Office. LMRO/H29/NF/Y/0/2/1–30.

Chapter 6

Life in Earlswood and the Reforms

The Earlswood medical advisors met on 1 September 1858[1] and reviewed the testimonials of the three applicants for the post of Medical Superintendent. They unanimously recommended that John Langdon Down be appointed at a salary of £400 per annum, with furnished apartments, gas and coals. It was agreed that the Medical Superintendent should attend all the meetings of the House Committee which had responsibility for the daily running of the institution. He would not however, attend the Board Meetings. Langdon Down was now in a turmoil. He accepted the appointment but immediately regretted it, probably because he had no relevant experience.

He wrote to his sister Sarah 'I have been very wretched the past week. The notion that I have made a great mistake haunts me day and night. I feel that by a strange combination of circumstances I was led into this and prevented consulting until too late, those who would have influenced me against it'. Mary Crellin may have suddenly realized that, if she were to marry him, she too would be committed to living in the Asylum; they were both afraid of the unknown. His sister tried her best to cheer him up and on the spur of the moment suggested that she and her husband go to Earlswood and look after his household needs until he found his feet. His sister too then had second thoughts and, not wishing to leave her home in London, urged him to review his engagement to Mary Crellin and marry her directly[2].

He seemed uncertain about his future though and was not yet ready for marriage. For one thing he still had examinations to take. His sister and her husband relented and moved to Earlswood. They spent a very unhappy winter there; amongst other things they found that the building was not properly heated. By misfortune there were also unduly large numbers of deaths among the patients. The Crellins paid for their board and also had the expense of hiring a horse and cab locally and on the carriage of their furniture to Earlswood. They had to do this because the hospital accommodation proved to be very sparsely furnished. In addition, they subsidized a stall at the annual bazaar.

Langdon Down was especially concerned about the prospect of bringing a new bride to live in the accommodation in Earlswood where they would share the building with its unsettled resident population. Mary visited frequently over the first year and was not deterred by what she saw. They must have had long and serious discussions but, having assessed the surroundings and the atmosphere in which they would live, finally made the decision to marry in the autumn of 1860.

He clearly had to find his feet before he could contemplate bringing a young wife into the rather austere and limited accommodation which had been made available to him. He also had examinations to take and wanted to commence his appointment as the holder of a university medical degree, as distinct from the Apothecaries Certificate which he held at the time of his appointment. His starting date at Earlswood was delayed accordingly. As an apothecary he would, according to the conventions of the time, have been known as Mr Down. With a medical degree he would be called Dr Down. He took up his post on 1 October, 1858.

During his first year in Earlswood, Langdon Down was still busy with his academic studies. Within the first year he took his MD degree in the University of London and the examination for Membership of the Royal College of Physicians. The latter, then as now, was a very searching examination, with a pass rate of only 25%. He was anxious to complete his programme of postgraduate studies before he married. His days were occupied with his medical and administrative duties and his nights in study. He threw himself enthusiastically into the improvement of the conditions in Earlswood.

He married Mary Crellin on 10 October 1860 at Mare Street Chapel in Hackney, according to the rites of the Baptist Church. The ceremony was conducted by the Reverend David Ford, who was married to Langdon Down's sister, Jane. John Langdon Down and Mary were both 31 years of age. The witnesses were Philip Crellin, Mary's father, her brother, Philip Crellin junior, John Rains, Mary's cousin and Henry Broadbent, a family friend. John Rains was to show family solidarity later when the Langdon Downs struck out on their own and needed financial backing in developing their own private institution. John Rain's sister, Eliza, was a close friend of Mary Crellin's and, in due course, her daughter Fanny became a daughter figure for the Langdon Downs. Fanny Rains was the one to rally to Mary's support in later years when Langdon Down died. Her letters to Mary always sparkled with warm affection and she addressed her always with familiarity as 'Dear Aunt', not as 'Aunt Mary', showing an easy intimacy. It was to be Fanny who rode with Mary in the first funeral carriage when Langdon Down was finally laid to rest.

In going into Earlswood, John Langdon Down had cause for anxiety. He went to Earlswood straight from medical school. Although he had been a brilliant student, he was completely new to the specialist field of learning disability and the associated problems and had no training in this field. He was breaking new ground and there was no body of knowledge he could draw on nor were there experts to give him orientation or instruction. There was noone to whom he could turn for advice on a daily basis.

He became close colleagues with Dr John Conolly and greatly looked forward to his monthly visits. Conolly kept up a voluntary connection with Earlswood throughout the whole period of Langdon Down's programme of reform. He wrote of Conolly; 'His visits were the most refreshing incidents of my recollection in connection with the asylum. Entering on my work as an untried man, and finding myself allied to an institution which had become unpopular at the Lunacy Board, I was mainly decided on holding a position which had so much to overwhelm one, by the influence of Dr Conolly. That influence was magical. The humility of his character was only equalled by the real love he manifested for the mentally afflicted'[3]. Langdon Down absorbed from him a philosophy of expectant optimism. John Conolly's optimism sustained him through the slow process of rehabilitating his patients. He found himself to be responsible for staff recruitment, the purchase of equipment and supplies, the organization of the pharmacy, the control of schools and workshops, and all of this in addition to the medical supervision. He entered on his duties without any prior experience of the problems involved.

Mary Crellin was a most compatible and supportive helpmate. Like Langdon Down she came from a deeply religious background. Her father Philip was an outfitter in Hackney and the family was fairly wealthy. She threw herself into the organization of activities and entertainments for the residents, frequently performing many duties herself. She became involved in the training programmes and, in due course, extended her work to include the supervision of residents who boarded with staff members and in other local houses, but who had not been formally admitted to Earlswood. This was an additional source of income but was to be a bone of contention with the Governors at a later stage.

Her husband's responsibilities extended into every area of management. A farm steward was appointed but he was not a member of the House Committee and it was left to the Medical Superintendent to report on foot rot among the sheep, the output of milk from the dairy herd, the timing of the harvest and all the other matters which arose in connection with the 150 acres which the Asylum ultimately acquired. For his sister Sarah, who had sacrificed so much to give him support, times had changed. When Langdon Down married she returned with her husband to her family home. She had supported John Langdon Down through all his academic life and shared with him all his successes. Now she found herself in a secondary role. The Crellins remained childless. To a degree, the loss of her status as the provider for an up and coming professional on the escalator of success had been taken

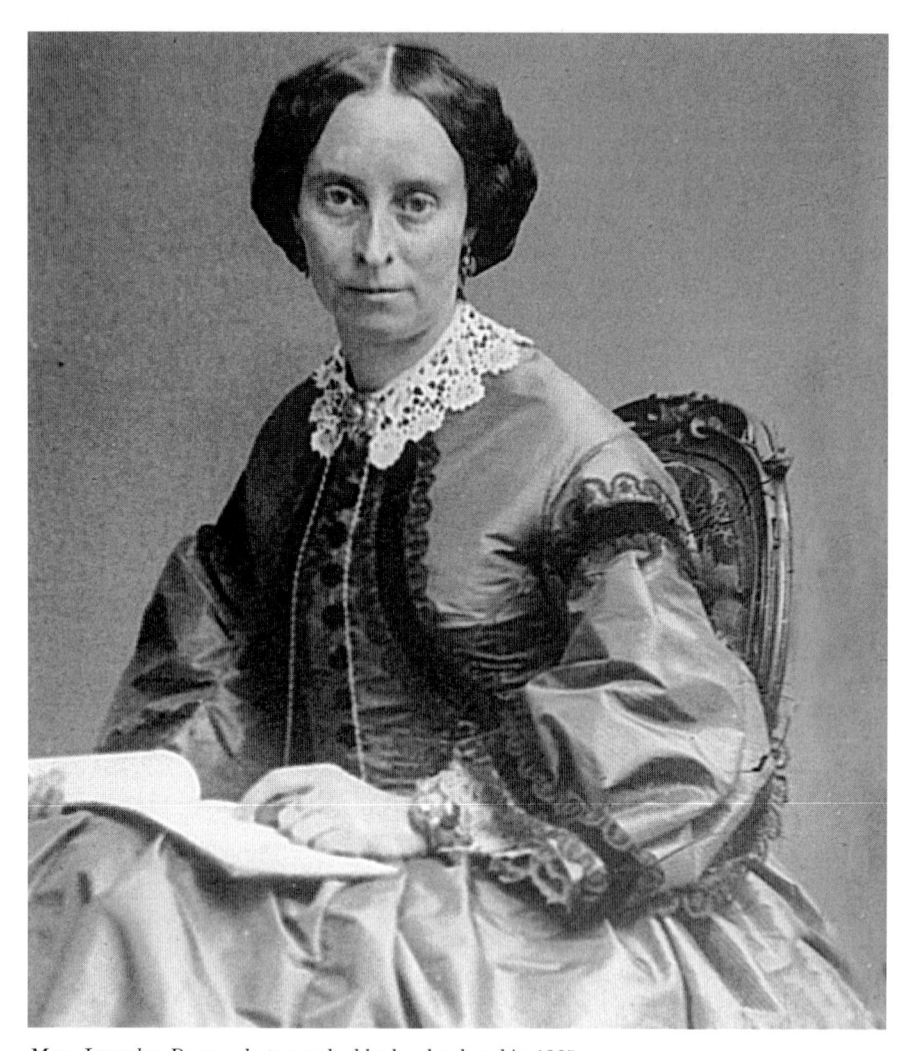

Mary Langdon Down, photographed by her husband in 1865.

away from her. Relations between the sisters-in-law remained uneasy and time did not heal the rift. Sarah felt excluded and after Langdon Down's death she wrote bitterly of 'the powers that be in the Langdon Down household in Normansfield'[1].

Langdon Down was, by temperament, a jovial extrovert. He never allowed his own extraordinary academic accomplishments to distance him from the less talented among his acquaintances. He had great empathy and was regarded with affection by everyone he worked with. When he came to leave Earlswood, having had a number of disagreements with the Hospital Board, the employees presented him with an elegant tea and coffee service, in testimony of their esteem and respect and this was accompanied by a suitable address.

When Charles Buxton, MP, visited Earlswood in 1864 he wrote to the Board to say: 'I feel that I ought not to conclude my remarks about the Asylum without saying that the Managers have, in Dr Down, the right man in the right place. I could not help being forcibly struck at the interest he took in all the inmates and the pleasure they experienced in seeing him as he accompanied me over the estate, coming round him as they did, and taking his hand and evincing their unfeigned delight in his presence[4]'. He inspired trust and affection and the Earlswood residents welcomed him with open arms.

Matilda J's family, whose child's disastrous outcome had, in part, led to Langdon Down's appointment, had accepted a payment of £250 in lieu of damages. Langdon Down's responsibility was to restore confidence in medical management. He devised training programmes aimed firstly at coordinating finger movements and then moving on to coordinate lip and tongue movements, on the clear understanding that until these were developed speech would necessarily remain impaired. He reviewed diets, making certain that they were well-balanced. He searched for ideas and, at the earliest possible opportunity, explored in-depth proposals for improvement put forward by the Commissioners in Lunacy. In March 1859 he reported that the Commissioners had devoted over eight hours to far-reaching discussions with him. He reported to the House Committee on the first steps that he had taken[5]. He felt that every aspect of living should contribute to education and wrote:

> I am of the opinion that giving proper food in proper measure will not accomplish all that we profess to do if some attention is not paid to the manner in which that food is partaken. I have given directions to the attendants to take pains in instructing [residents] in the proper use of the knife and fork etc. and to regard the general arrangements at table as part of the educational system. But with respect to the meals of breakfast and tea, I have always felt ashamed for visitors to see what was literally our process of feeding; the beverage, supplied in tin cups, rudely dipped by hand into large jugs, and the bread and butter coarsely cut and handed round and placed in unseemly piles on the bare greasy cloth. Some of the freshly admitted cases, I know, have been sensitive enough to feel the humiliation of their new position. I have, as far as our store would allow, in the past week used cups and saucers. Plates are being supplied to all. The present system of dipping should be replaced by metal teapots of large size and the bread should be supplied in weighed rolls. I feel that in the management of our pupils we lose an important aid for their elevation and improvement whenever we disregard the amenities of life[5].

In his approach to staffing levels, his attitude was that quality was more important than quantity. In a series of steps he set about reducing staff numbers and improving efficiency. He wrote on 4th April, 1859, that he had made considerable alterations to the domestic arrangements. Early on he formed the opinion that the conduct of the institution was too expensively managed, arising from the employment of too many people. This appeared to have arisen from three causes; the late rising on the part of domestic staff, the best part of the day being wasted by the long lunches which dragged on without control and the mistaken policy of employing two inefficient persons at low salaries instead of one competent person on a fair salary. The latter policy also disregarded the fact that the cost of boarding two was double that of boarding one.

He entirely abolished the custom of staggered lunches. In order to effect this the dinner of the staff was scheduled for 1.15 pm, the pupils to dine at 12.30 pm. He abolished what he regarded as the evil custom of supplying individual servants' rations to the pupils, allowing them to take their meals when and how they pleased. 'Every cupboard throughout the building was in a filthy state of confusion and the bedrooms the scenes of luncheons and evening meals. These irregularities have been abolished by the serving out of rations in bulk for the entire servant staff and requiring that every servant in the establishment have all their meals in the dining hall[6]'. He was concerned at the low level of wages and, in order to change this, colluded with the Commissions in Lunacy. With appropriate prompting, the Commissioners asked for a list of the staff members and the wages and duties of each. The reductions in staff numbers he recommended were planned to reduce the annual wage bill by £200 (£12,000 at present value).

He introduced an upward system of graduation for the residents; 'I have arranged that some of the worst cases should no longer be brought in to the dining hall, but should have their meals in a separate room where they can have all the attention their peculiarities require, and at the same time preserving the peace of the major part of the family'[7]. The residents were always referred to as 'the family'. From January 1859, he was made responsible for approving every staff appointment. He also secured the approval of the House Committee to the conduct of postmortem examinations, which should be made in all cases where this was possible. Over the next decade, he carried out the postmortems himself and his search for a scientific basis for learning disability continued. He acquired very extensive experience. In his second Lettsomian lecture of 1887 he wrote of having seen 2000 patients.

By 1861 he had carried out 100 postmortem examinations on the brains of Earlswood patients and by 1866 this number had risen to 150. When he left Earlswood he bought his own microscope to use in Normansfield, his next institution. In doing postmortems he removed the vault of the skull carefully to measure in detail and to compare it with the adjacent brain structure. He took photographs of some of the brains that he examined, one of which has survived. Eight of his skull specimens went with him from Earlswood to Normansfield and have remained there. Unfortunately, the patients concerned are not identified.

It is interesting that, in spite of his growing experience of postmortem examination, Langdon Down did not refer in his published work to any structural changes in the brains of his 'Mongolian' patients. However, the state of medical knowledge of the age in which he lived meant his failure to identify the rather unobtrusive evidence of change in brain structure was shared by all other observers. Fraser and Mitchell, in 1876, went no further than suggesting slightly deficient development of some parts of the brain surface[8]. It was not until 1908 that Hill, in his paper on 'Mongolism and its Pathology', clearly identified a structural abnormality[9]. Langdon Down was a clinician. Detailed structural change could only be recognized by a trained professional and, in the 1850s, there were no professional pathologists. It is to Langdon Down's credit that he pursued the question of postmortem examination so vigorously in spite of the heavy workload which he also carried. He received no extra remuneration for these extra duties, but the attendant who assisted him at the postmortems was given an increase of £3 in his annual salary because of the unpleasant nature of his duties, moving up from £25 per annum to £28.

In spite of his easy manner Langdon Down was a disciplinarian. An unnamed basket-maker who was not considered efficient was discharged and another one sought[10]. An assistant master called Snell had been noted to develop the habit of appropriating scuttles of coal from the school room for his own private apartment. Mr Snell's schoolroom pass key was taken from him and he later resigned from the Institution[11]. Langdon Down's directives to the staff barred punishments of all kinds.

Years later, in his third Lettsomian lecture, he set out his views. He said of the care of the patient:

> While his physical and mental powers are being developed by hygienic and physiological processes, he has to be taught to subordinate his will to that of another. He has to learn obedience: that right-doing brings pleasure, and that wrong-doing is followed by its deprivation. The effective faculties should be so cultivated that the deprivation of the love of the teacher should be the greatest punishment and that its manifestation the highest reward. In this way indications of untruthfulness, selfishness, obstinacy, sensuality, theft and unkindness to companions are checked. Corporal punishment should be strictly forbidden. The tact of the teacher will be called in to exercise in devising a

suitable reward or punishment. I have seen a girl exhibiting violent obstinacy melted into contrition and obedience by the threat of the teacher that she would wipe away from her face the kiss that she had given her the previous day. In no case should the punishment interfere with the hygienic treatment. Nothing is worse than the deprivation of food for an offence. I have seen a case of violent and uncontrollable temper reduced to calm obedience by the administration of a basin of bread and milk[12].

Langdon Down had an anxiety about abuse of the beer ration which was supplied to attendants. Until he had been appointed, beer had been made available, without control, to both staff and patients. His predecessor, Dr Maxwell, had agreed to increasing the attendants' ration to two pints a day. Langdon Down's first step was to reduce this allowance to one pint a day. He later arranged that beer should be made available to individual patients on a named basis only. The supply of beer to patients was to be vouched for by the Medical Superintendent himself. By contrast the allowance of port to the Board, purchased for the refreshment of its members at the monthly meeting went unchallenged, and three dozen bottles of good port were purchased for their comfort. He tempered his reforming zeal with discretion[13]. He ventured into the area of supplies and purchasing. He recommended that the quality of meat would be better and cheaper if whole sheep were bought and then butchered. He was required by the Board to follow up complaints and indeed in his first month in post he was requested by the Board to attend to the quality of the potatoes, because they were not as good as they should be.

The Commissioners in Lunacy had frequently expressed concern about the failure of the Asylum to maintain the statutory medical records, recording the progress of each individual patient. Once again, Langdon Down got on with the business and by 1860 the Commissioners reported that the medical visitation book was properly and carefully kept[14]. The Commissioners in Lunacy reported as follows: 'We have the satisfaction of being enabled to report most favourably on the personal condition of the pupils and the continued good arrangement of the Institution by the Superintendent, Matron and other officers. The pupils were, without exception, cheerful, happy, well-dressed and clean and neat in their persons. The medical visitation book is now properly and carefully kept'.

They also reported that the Institution generally exhibited marked improvement. Langdon Down had clearly stimulated the House Committee into greater activity. The Commissioners learnt with much satisfaction that the House Committee were now making regular and frequent visits and that the system of management had been progressively improved by greater attention being paid to the physical and industrial development of the intellectual faculties, however feeble, by such natural means in preference to attempting to accomplish too much by mental instruction in school. The committee had been concerned at adverse publicity in the press. Mr Boyle St John of the *Telegraph* newspaper was invited to visit and toured the asylum with the members. After full inspection he expressed himself much pleased with all that he had seen[15]. The problem with the press did not recur. Throughout the whole of 1858 and for the first year of John Langdon Down's appointment, John Conolly took the chair at the meetings of the House Committee. His fatherly presence helped and supported John Langdon Down in settling into his job, both socially and professionally.

The Commissioners in Lunacy had supported the concept of paying a sufficiently high salary to the Superintendent to attract an efficient and competent officer. In addition they had previously expressed the opinion that Langdon Down's predecessor had never had sufficient power and they considered that his successor should have full control, not only over the other officers and servants, but also over the general management of the establishment. In addition he should publish a report annually on the general condition of the hospital. When Langdon Down was in post they reinforced this view and reported that they were glad to learn that, in his capacity of Medical Superintendent, he was admitted to be present at some meetings of the Board. Also, as the responsible head of the institution, he was invested with adequate authority to carry out the system of management which he considered conducive to its usefulness and efficiency.

The problem of wet and dirty beds was taken in hand by tightening up on the supervision of night staff. Clocks were introduced to ensure that attendants lifted those children who needed it. The night attendants, called the night watch, woke each pupil of 'uncleanly habits' three times in the night by clapping their hands. It was noted that children went back to sleep again immediately after being lifted, their rest being practically unbroken. By 1861 the Commissioners found that there were only four dirty beds and fifteen wet beds the night before they visited.

Langdon Down received further experience in management strategy when he became involved in the sinking of a well in the search for better water supplies. When he was first appointed the water was drawn from a brook. It was often turbid and discoloured and of bad taste. The well was expected to yield a good supply of water at 300 feet but failed to do so. Boring continued down to 500 feet with disappointing results. When the bore hole reached a depth of 920 feet a daily output of only 1300 gallons was obtained. This was enough for drinking and cooking but an additional 3000 gallons a day had to be bought from the British Land Company before the problem

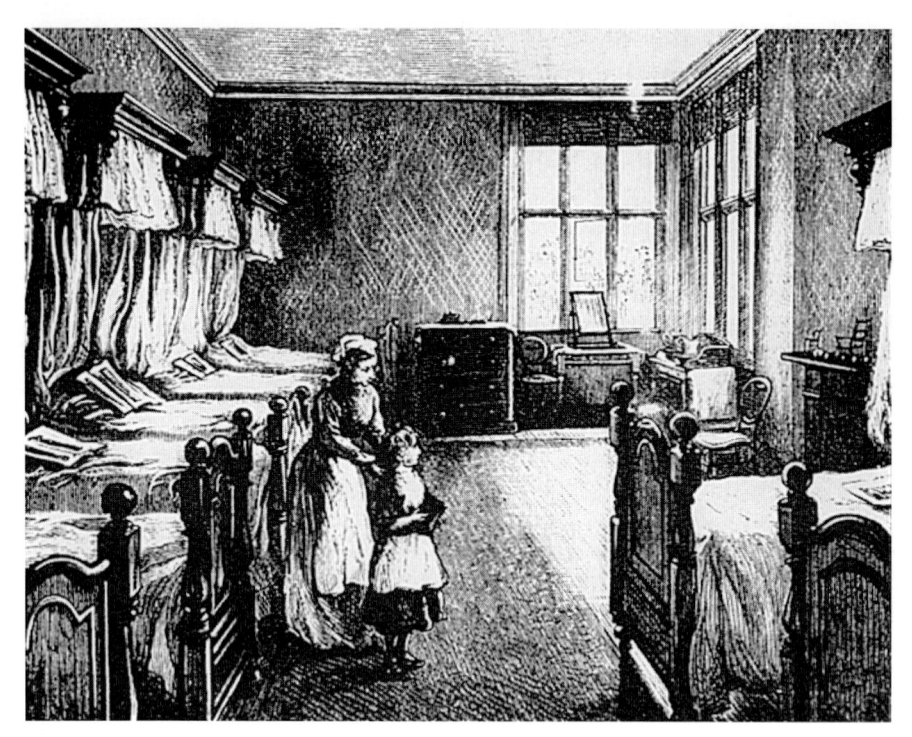

An Earlswood dormitory, 1880.

was solved. Langdon Down was kept busy with analytical reports, surveyors' reports and engineers' reports. Professor Austin was called in consultation. He advised drilling no further. The total cost had been £1800 (£108,000 at present values). Langdon Down must have been pleased to see the end of the project.

At the time of his appointment Langdon Down had responsibility for 207 patients. By 1865 the number had increased to 418. It was not until 1865 that steps were taken to recruit an assistant medical officer, the salary offered being £100 per annum (£6,000 at present value). A schoolmaster, assistant master, school mistress and assistant were employed and, with the assistance of interested attendants, two-thirds of the children were formally taught in school rooms. They had 10 teaching hours a week and were graded in six classes, from children who could read fairly well, through to those who could not read at all. The emphasis in the school was on the practical understanding of simple reading and arithmetic for practical applications, such as shopping.

Extensive workshops were built and the boys who showed potential competence were taught carpentry, tailoring, shoemaking, mat-making, basket-making, plumbing, farming, gardening and housework. The girls were taught household duties and needlework. The staffing ratio – including attendants, servants, teachers and nurses – was one care worker for every three residents. Approximately half the residents on the school roll attended for a whole day, and half for the morning only. In 1861 Miss Fagg, the head teacher, reported that only a few of the children could read the Bible. She concentrated on teaching by what she described as the infant system, combining amusement with instruction, physical effort with mental exercise and an overall concentration on mental exercises to develop and strengthen the faculties of the children. She was devoted to 'my afflicted children', and hoped that she would be able to continue devoting her energies to improving their unfortunate condition as much as possible. She worked closely with Langdon Down; when he eventually left in 1868 relationships with the Board broke down and Miss Fagg ended up being dismissed.

In 1865 the Institution was virtually self-sufficient. It had its own bakery and laundry and all footwear was made in the workshops. The farm supplied all the fruit and vegetables required. The sewage of the Asylum was distributed over the grass on the farm and even during a very dry summer there was enough milk from the Asylum's herd. This pattern of self-sufficiency was one that Langdon Down was later to try and emulate in his own private institution in Normansfield. The Commissioners were anxious to see residents involved in laundry work but Langdon Down was slow to agree. He may have been concerned about the possibility of an accident and, indeed, in 1868 an inquest was held on a boy who was accidentally scalded to death in a bath. The safety key which was used to control each hot water tap had gone missing and an accident occurred.

Morning and evening prayers were said in the dining hall, which was used as an assembly room. On Sundays church service was conducted and in 1862 the Commissioners in Lunacy reported that 300 residents attended Sunday morning church service[16]. The residents were reported to show much interest in the religious exercises and it was considered that these had a good effect on them. A barrel organ had been brought into service and the children enjoyed the music. In addition, 100 children went out once a month to a special service in a nearby church. The Commissioners continued to look forward to the time when the funds at the disposal of the Asylum would enable it to provide a chapel for Divine Worship and, at various times, suggested that a chaplain should be appointed; however this never occurred during the time that Langdon Down was Superintendent.

There was continuing interest in the progress of those discharged. In 1862 Langdon Down reported to the Commissioners that 29 out of 31 were considered to be improved to some degree, 17 were improved, the majority of these greatly improved, and 12 had profited so much that they were able to work for a livelihood[16]. Some had secured regular employment, the girls in domestic service and the boys as carpenters, tailors and mat-makers. A great deal of valuable information concerning the Earlswood residents has been assembled by Dr David Wright. He has analysed the backgrounds of patients, their mode of admission and duration of stay, the institution's finances and its recruitment policies. His unsympathetic evaluation of Langdon Down is referred to in Chapter 8[17].

Visitors came from far and wide to see Earlswood; the visitors book has signatures from Sweden, Germany, Holland and the US as well as from all parts of the British Isles. Cheyne Brady visited and wrote afterwards from Dublin with great enthusiasm, describing Langdon Down as able and intelligent. He saw all the workshops in action and the special training in simple skills such as dressing and undressing, as well as the more advanced teaching of shopping skills. He also heard the Earlswood band play and said that all the instruments were played by employees except the drum, which was played by an idiot savant. Langdon Down, he said, enjoyed the unmistakeable affection of the children. He described Earlswood as unique and said he had never had such a happy day[18].

References

1 Unpublished correspondence, courtesy of Lord Christopher Brain. Undated letter of Sarah Crellin, 1896.
2 Unpublished correspondence, courtesy of Lord Christopher Brain.
3 Clark J. *A Memoir of John Conolly*. London: John Murray, 1869: 118–20.
4 Surrey Record Office. SRO;392/1/2/1. Letters.
5 Surrey Record Office. SRO;392/3/1/3. Medical Superintendent's Report to the House Committee.
6 Surrey Record Office. SRO;392/3/1/ 3F243. House Committee.
7 Surrey Record Office. SRO;392/3/1/ 3F258. House Committee.
8 Fraser J, Mitchell A. Kalmuc Idiocy; report of a case with autopsy. *J Ment Sc* 1876; **22**: 169–79.
9 Hill WB. Mongolism and its pathology. *Quart J Med* 1908; **2**: 49–68.
10 Surrey Record Office. SRO;392/3/1/3. House Committee.
11 Surrey Record Office. SRO;392/2/1/6/F262. Letters.
12 *Mental Affections of Childhood and Youth*. Churchill, 1887: 139.
13 Surrey Record Office. SRO;392/3/1/3, F186. House Committee.
14 Surrey Record Office. SRO;392/10/1/1. Commissioner's Report, 1860.
15 Surrey Record Office. SRO;392/3/1/3. House Committee.
16 Surrey Record Office. SRO;392/10/1/1. Commissioner's Report, 1962.
17 Wright D. *The National Asylum for Idiots, Earlswood, 1847–86*. Unpublished PhD Thesis University of Oxford, 1993.
18 Brady C. *The Training of Idiotic and Feeble-minded Children*. Dublin: Hodges Smith, 1865.

Chapter 7

Family Affairs

Apart from a very heavy clinical case-load and the responsibility of dealing with an ever increasing number of feeble and disorganized residents, Langdon Down set about the daunting task of providing better services for education, vocational training, physical development, entertainment and religious instruction. His concepts were set out by him in his address to the Social Science Congress, published under the title *Education and Training of the Feeble in Mind*[1]. He also set them out in his contribution to Quain's *Dictionary of Medicine* in 1882[2]. The patient, he said,

> ...should be rescued from his solitary life and have the companionship of his peers. He should be surrounded by influences both of art and nature, calculated to make his life joyous, to arouse his observation and to quicken his power of thought...success can only be obtained by keeping the patient in the highest possible health. Diet should be liberal...The rooms he inhabits should be well ventilated whilst kept warm: and daily baths with shampooing should be employed. Of first importance is the soil; a clay soil is fatal to all proper progress inducing tuberculosis and lowering the vital power. Physical training forms an important part of the treatment. The attenuated muscles have to be nourished by calling into exercise their functions and the automatic and rhythmic movements have to be replaced by others which are the product of the will. The training has to be carried out in minute detail...The moral education is of paramount importance. The pupil has to be taught to subordinate his will to that of another. He has to learn obedience, that right doing is productive of pleasure and that wrongdoing is followed by deprivation thereof...The intellectual training must be based on the cultivation of the senses. The patient should be taught the qualities, form and relation of objects by their sense of touch: to apprehend colour, size, number, shape and relation by sight: to understand the varieties of sound that address the ear: the qualities of objects by taste and smell. These lessons should be of the simplest at first, gradually accumulative. Nothing should be left to the imagination. The idiot must be taught the concrete and not the abstract...He should be taught to dress and undress himself, to acquire habits of order and neatness, to use the spoon or knife and fork, to walk with precision, to handle with tact. The

defective speech is best overcome by a well arranged plan of tongue gymnastics, followed by cultivation of the purely imitative powers[1].

He had quickly noted among the residents a great fondness for music and found that simple airs were often readily learned. He set about taking advantage of this. In the days before radio and television, entertainment had to be a home-grown product. Formal concerts were held monthly and there were weekly rehearsals. By 1865 recruitment from among members of staff had brought into being a brass band and an orchestra. A grand piano was donated and an appeal launched among the friends of the payment cases raised most of the money to purchase an organ[3]. The Coldstream Guards also donated a bassoon.

He tried to prepare his young people for life in the outside world. Visitors commented favourably on the way in which he had set up shopkeeping lessons[4]. Some children acted as buyers and some as sellers of common objects, all at the same time being instructed clearly in the elements of knowledge concerning money, numbers and weights and measures. The schoolmaster was encouraged in giving attention to speech. Croquet, aunt Sally and a game called white, red and blue were introduced. Cricket matches were played on Wednesdays and Saturdays by teams made up of members of staff. Over a mile of continuous walks were developed within the grounds and a plantation of 6000 forest trees was laid down, with winding roads and paths leading through every part of it. In the dining room a member of staff sat at the head of each table. Before each meal the residents rose and, with their hands behind their backs, sang grace before and after meals, which the Commissioners reported in 1869 was conducted in a very satisfactory manner. The only bone of contention with the Commissioners with respect to the diet was that beer was not allowed and, on several occasions over the years they expressed the view that 'considering the low state of vitality and the prevalence of chilblains, we strongly recommend that it should be a part of the ordinary diet'. Langdon Down demurred. His attitudes softened as he grew older and he came, in time, to preside at well-fuelled medical functions and to prudently savour the fruit of the vine.

The hope that the residents would benefit from education and training led to a concentration on early admission. The 1863 annual report[5] set out that:

> ...persons in poor circumstances, especially in the labouring classes...are content to bear the burden of maintenance until they attain the age of 14–15 years, partly no doubt with the hope of becoming able to assist in gaining a living, and they postponed all attempts to get better care so that it is only when a neglected

boy or girl is found growing up mischievous or dangerous that they become anxious to be relieved of the trouble and expense. This delay has a tendency to gradually fill the Asylum with troublesome young men and women brought up with no kind of wholesome restraint...when young children (5–7) have been received into the Asylum, their progress generally has been satisfactory[5].

The Board therefore decided to encourage early admission limiting the upper age for application for the first admission to 12 years.

The Asylum began to derive a small income from the workshops and, in 1862, a profit of £150 was made on handiwork. Each year new entertainments were introduced. There were visits from a Punch and Judy show, charades set against scenery, croquet – which in the circumstances may have seemed a little hazardous – donkey cart rides and each year a visit by 100 of the residents to Crystal Palace.

There was a continuous process of upgrading the quality of recruitment, which was personally undertaken by Langdon Down. He negotiated increases in salaries and by 1868 nurses, who might in the past have started with annual salaries as low as £6 per annum, now started at £14 with annual increments up to £18 (£1000 today). Attendants who formerly started at £20 now started at £25, with annual increases up to £30. These scales must be looked at in relation to annual incomes in general at that time; for example, unskilled workers in 1867 had annual incomes of £47, skilled manual workers £86 and house maids £10 increasing to £14[6]. It is difficult to quantify the value of board and lodging but it must have been worth about £1 per week. The increases in salaries and wages were clearly necessary but, once they had been awarded and taking into account the value of board and lodging, they brought the scales into alignment with the accepted norms of the day.

In his personal life Langdon Down, with the last of his examinations out of the way and newly married, found that his wife became a major support in his professional as well as domestic life. She organized and participated in entertainments and indeed their joint experience of these led to the continuing use of drama as a therapeutic exercise in their own establishment at Normansfield in due course. In 1862 their first baby was on the way. He asked that the secretary's office be given up to him as an additional bedroom. The Chairman, Mr Abbiss, subsequently reported back to the House Committee on his further discussions with the Medical Superintendent and recommended that the House Committee be requested to provide Dr Down with an alternative extra sleeping room. A nurse's sitting room was converted into a bedroom for the family.

Their first child was a boy, born in 1862. They chose the name Everleigh, a name which was new to the family. His proud father photographed him as an infant and again as a little boy of three or four years, attired as little boys were in those days in a ribboned dress. Everleigh was to die tragically at the age of 21 years and little is known about him.

Lilian, the only daughter of the Langdon Downs, was born in 1863. Her photograph at the age of two shows a sturdy, fair-haired, bright-eyed girl, her hair braided and in a pretty dress. In the year in which she had her photograph taken she was devastated by illness. She developed a high temperature with convulsive seizures; this is not infrequent in children but Lilian's did not follow the usual course. Instead of subsiding quickly within minutes, as feverish convulsions usually do, her seizures continued intermittently over a

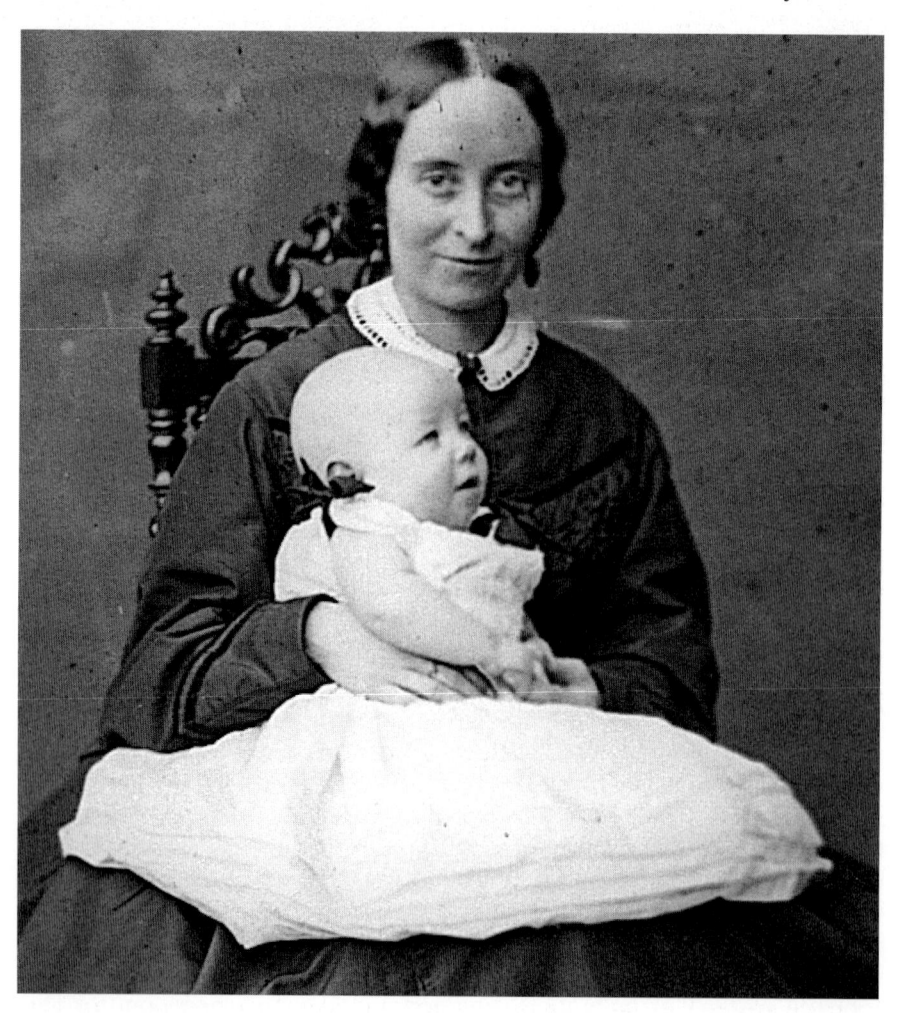

Mary with her first child, Everleigh, born in 1862.

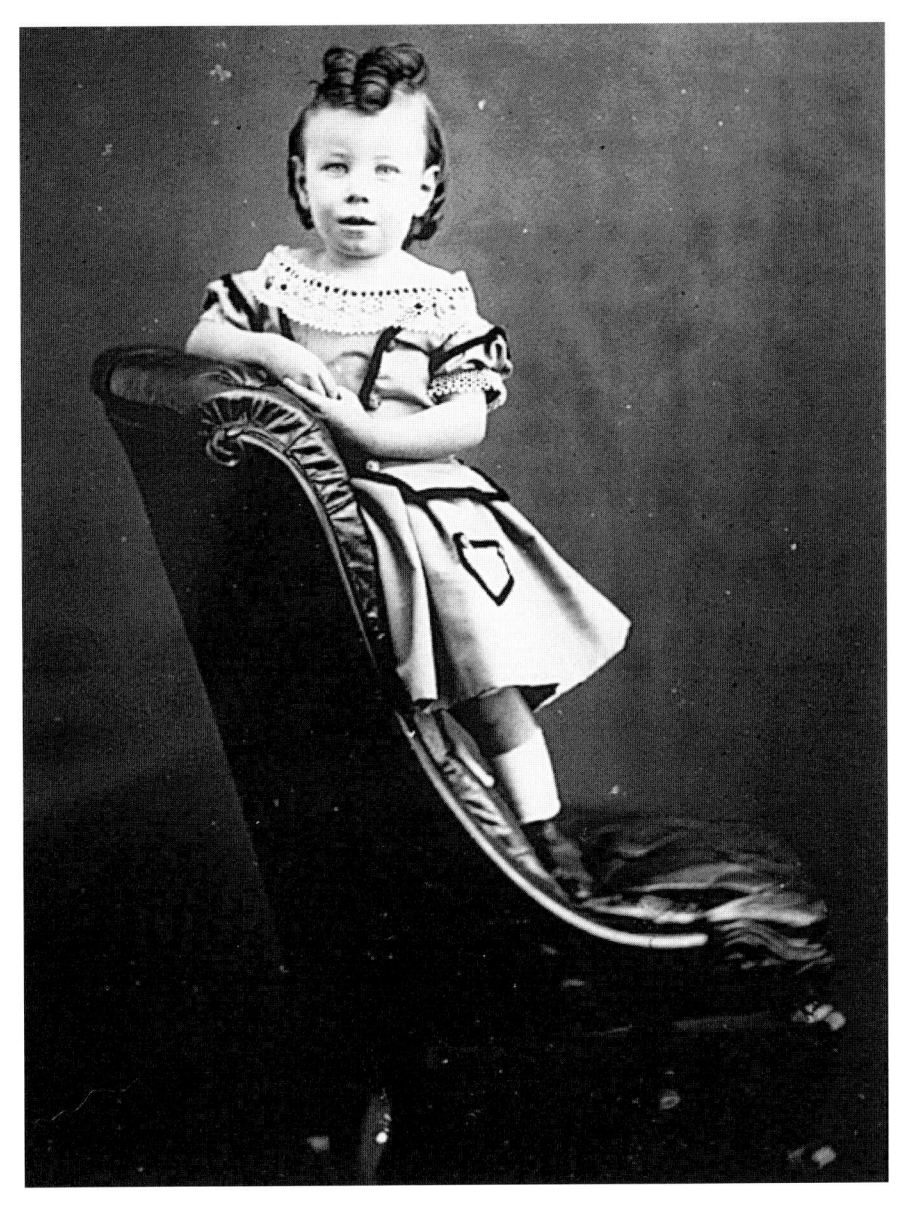

Everleigh, aged four years, dressed according to the prevailing custom. Boys did not wear trousers until at least the age of five years.

period of several days. Presumably she had a viral brain infection. If it had been a straightforward case of bacterial meningitis, her father would have known, but even if he did there was no anti-bacterial treatment which could have saved her.

She lingered on for two weeks before she died. Her death was a terrible blow. Her parents purchased a grave in the Nonconformist plot in Reigate cemetery. Her mother was distraught but searched

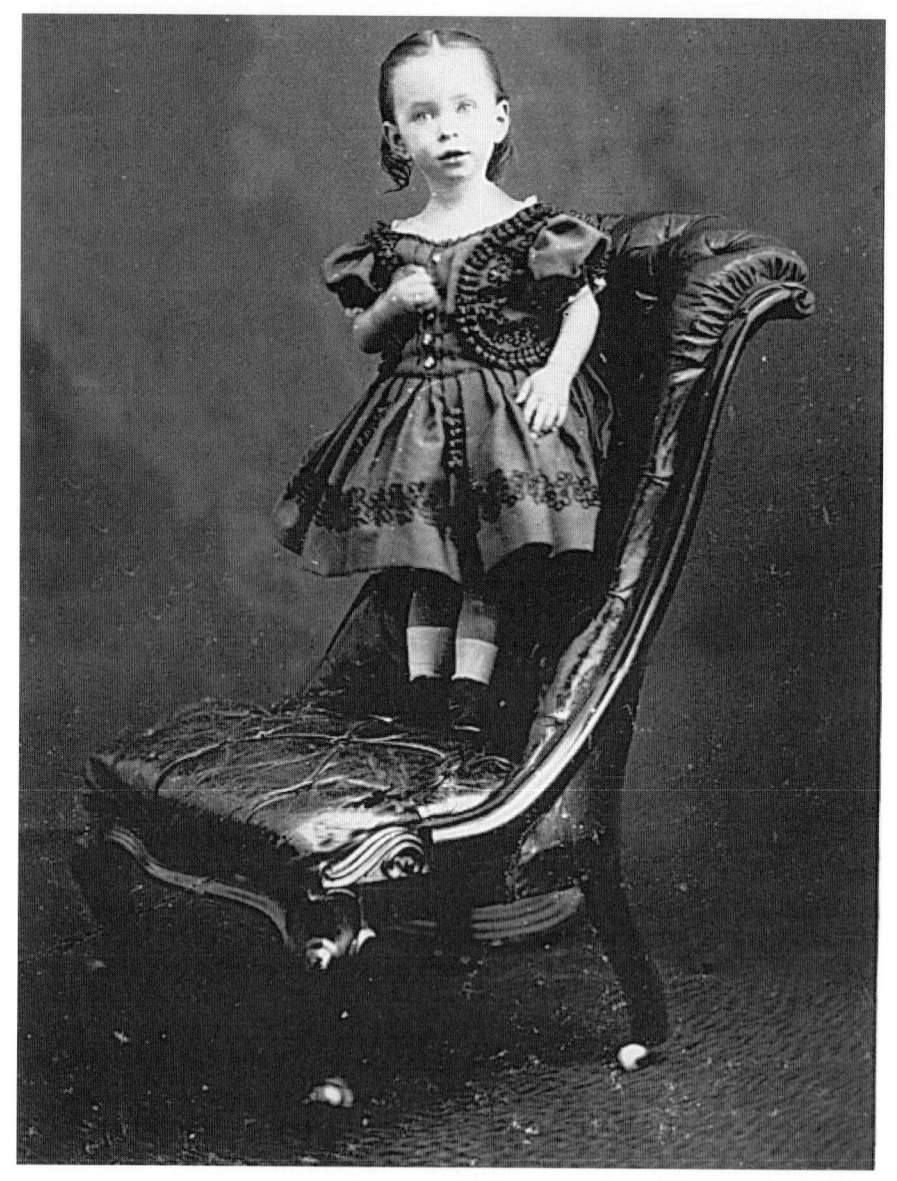

Lilian, the Langdon Downs' only daughter, aged two. Photographed by her father in the year she died.

for words for a tombstone inscription. Her final choice was short and simple: 'Happy soul to the sight of Jesus gone'. Other choices penned and discarded by her distressed mother were all of a similar religious orientation, such as: 'He shall gather the lambs to Him', or 'Jesus called a little child unto Him' [Unpublished correspondence]. Mary Langdon Down held these thoughts dear to her. When Everleigh, the eldest son, was buried in 1873 in the same plot, his mother looked again at the list of possible inscriptions and for Everleigh she chose the last in the original list she had drawn up for Lilian: 'Until the daybreak and the shadows flee away'.

Mary suffered intensely. She became very ill and this may have been a reactive depression. In 1863 there had been a major epidemic of scarlet fever in the Royal Earlswood Asylum. It is possible that sporadic cases still occurred in 1864 and she may have been a victim of this. Likewise there were occasional cases of typhoid fever. After Lilian's death Mary put her pen to paper and wrote a very touching poem, full of a mother's grief but firmly expressing the hope of resurrection and reunion.

She prefaces the poem she wrote with a quotation from St Matthew's Gospel, 18:10, 'Take heed that ye despise not one of these little ones; for I say unto you that in heaven these angels do always behold the face of my father which is in heaven'. The poem has survived in the family papers and is quoted with permission:

>A little precious babe
>Came to my heart one day
>And folded there most lovingly,
>A long sweet time she lay.
>
>Her little fairy fingers
>O'er my bosom softly crept
>A faint thrill ever lingers
>There where her pure cheek slept
>
>Her eyes were dark and beautiful
>As evening's starry sky
>Her voice as clear and musical
>As birds' that sing on high
>
>Like lilies gleamed her snowy skin
>Like pale gold shone her hair
>Like pearls, her rosy lips within
>Shone tiny teeth so fair
>
>So fair, so pure my little gem
>That angels came to see
>And seeing, bore her home with them
>Their angel babe to be
>
>And ever when cast down apart
>In agony I weep
>There thrills within my stricken heart
>A thought that ne'er shall sleep

That cradled in an angel's arm
From every sorrow free
A little bright winged seraph child
Waits lovingly for me

References

1. Langdon Down J. *The Education and Training of the Feeble in Mind*. London: Lewis, 1874.
2. Quain R. *Dictionary of Medicine*. London: Longmans, 1882.
3. Surrey Record Office. SRO;392/1/2/1. Annual Report, 1862.
4. Brady C. *The Training of Idiotic and Feeble-minded Children*. Dublin: Hodges and Smith, 1865.
5. Surrey Record Office. SRO;|392/1/2/1. Annual Report, 1863.
6. Bedarida F. *Social History of England 1851–1875*. Methuen, 1979.

Chapter 8

Dealing and Doctoring in Earlswood

Langdon Down met regularly with his colleagues in the London Hospital and knew that successful doctors could command high incomes. He had started in 1858 on a salary of £400 per annum (£24,000 today). In December 1861 the Board agreed that, in consideration of the highly satisfactory manner in which he had performed the duties of Physician and Superintendent and for the great interest he took in everything which concerned its welfare, the Board had much pleasure in increasing his salary to £500. They felt however, that it was only right that Dr Down should be informed that they made the advance to him in the hope that he would pledge himself to give the whole of his time to the services of the charity and take no further office with the London Hospital than he held at the time. He had gone to Earlswood with a part-time lectureship in comparative anatomy and, in 1859, had been appointed Assistant Physician at the London Hospital. In 1863 the secretary reported that Alderman Abbiss, the Chairman of the Board, had called to say that he had received a most important communication from Dr Down[1]. Langdon Down's letter of March 3 read as follows:

My Dear Sir,

When the Board made you the medium of communication with me in November 1861 in reference to the increase of my salary to £500 per annum, you were pleased to ask me not to take any steps which would remove me from Earlswood without communicating the nature of the circumstances through you to them.

In compliance with that request I have to inform you that in consequence of projected changes at the London Hospital, I have been offered the Chair of Physiology and have been informed that a more intimate connection with the Hospital is not far distant; a connection which, while increasing my status there would be incompatible with prolonged residence at Earlswood.

In fact I am called upon to elect my future course; I shall have either to resign my London Hospital appointment and decline the Chair of Physiology or to dissolve my connection with Earlswood. An important element in my decision is, of course, a pecuniary one and one which the Board alone can supply. May I therefore beg you to lay this communication before them and ask them if they would kindly indicate as nearly as possible what my future position at Earlswood is likely to be.

I am, my dear Sir,

Yours faithfully,

J Langdon H Down[1]

It was agreed to call a special Board Meeting for the following Wednesday. At the meeting on 11 March, Alderman Abbiss reported on the contents of Langdon Down's letter. He also said that it had come to his notice that Dr Little was about to resign his appointment as Physician at the London Hospital. It was necessary that Dr Down should shortly determine which course to adopt as, if he now declined to accept the offer, his connection with the London Hospital would for ever be severed and he was therefore anxious to learn what his future position at Earlswood was likely to be.

Abbiss asked Langdon Down to write to him with some idea of the future emoluments he would look to; a letter embodying these had been received and subsequently followed by another. In the second letter Dr Down expressed hope that the Board would not consider his first letter as dictating terms to them, but as a private letter to Alderman Abbiss, as he preferred to leave the matter in the hands of the Board. It was agreed to hold a special meeting and, in deference to Dr Down, to treat his letters as private. The matter was then fully ventilated and each member of the Board gave his opinion. The Board felt that they should not stand in the way of Dr Down's advancement in his profession, or be the means of affecting his future position and they would prefer the first action in the matter to be taken by Dr Down.

It was unanimously agreed that, although the Board were very desirous to retain the valuable services of Dr Down, they felt that in the present position of the charity they would not be justified in increasing the emoluments of the office of Resident Physician. On 15 April, Langdon Down replied to say that he had come to the conclusion not to sever his connection with the Institution and to remain at Earlswood. He requested an increase in fringe benefits. The letter was to be acknowledged and the points in it to be considered at the next Board Meeting. At a meeting on 17 June, it was proposed that he be supplied with butter, milk, eggs and vegetables at the expense of the Asylum but at a further meeting on 1 July, it was agreed that the subject be deferred. The Board had other steps in mind.

Langdon Down's approach to Alderman Abbiss is perplexing. The vacancy in physiology had arisen as a replacement for a Dr Andrew Clark. Andrew Clark had been appointed to a salaried lectureship in

1853 with a view to getting the medical museum exhibits well-arranged and catalogued. He had been paid a salary of £375 per annum and the hope was that the museum collection would be on a par with those of St Bartholomew's Hospital and of the Royal College of Surgeons. In April 1856 he had been appointed Lecturer in Physiology, having been given a strong assurance that the duties would not interfere with those of the curatorship of the museum.

In 1859 Andrew Clark had written to the London Hospital Medical Council to say that he greatly regretted that he had permitted attention to other and less important duties to interfere with the continuation and completion of the catalogue and that he offered to continue as an honorary unpaid officer of the Medical School, on the understanding that he would complete the catalogue. He was given until September 1859 to do this and his salary continued to be paid. The Medical School remained patient until three years later but, in December 1862, they passed a resolution requiring him to produce the catalogue at the next meeting. He replied on 17 December:

> I am carried to the conclusion that no alternative is left to me but to bring my official relations to the Council, now so peculiarly painful, to a close. I beg therefore, respectfully, to resign into the hands of the Council the appointment of Curator of the Museum and Lecturer in Physiology which I hold under its authority and I shall continue to hold until the appointment of a successor. I still hold myself responsible to the Council for the catalogue and I respectfully hope that so long as the work is progressing in a degree compatible with my health, I may be spared the extreme pain and humiliation of objurgatory resolutions[2].

Andrew Clark had ignored one of the basic rules of administration. In tendering his resignation he had put himself in a situation in which it might be accepted. The Council met on 27 October, accepted his resignation and proceeded to fill the vacancy. This is the point at which one can only assume that Dr Little, John Langdon Down's friend and admirer, approached him privately and endeavoured to head-hunt him for the post. No formal authority had been given to him but it would not have been unusual for informal discussions to have occurred and indeed the Council proceeded to make an appropriate arrangement, apparently without advertising the vacancy. On 22 June the Council, having probably been privately informed that Langdon Down was not a candidate, proceeded to make a joint appointment between Dr John Cooper and Dr Hughlings Jackson as joint Lecturers in Physiology.

Langdon Down had put in his request to Earlswood for an increase in salary but had agreed to defer it until the financial status of the Asylum had improved. Things happened quite quickly and, in 1865, his salary was increased to £600 per annum, backdated to December 1864 and to be increased by £50 per annum up to £700. This indeed equated to £42,000 today, which might be considered to be almost appropriate at the present time, taking into account the accommodation package and lower taxation rates of the era.

Additionally, he got formal sanction for absence from the hospital twice a week, so that he could attend to his duties at the London Hospital. He had so arranged these that he could undertake both his outpatient sessions, teaching sessions and Earlswood recruitment sessions on the same days. The Board of Earlswood was, however, anxious that these concessions should not be abused and he was required to keep an attendance book showing the days and times of his leaving and returning to the asylum[3]. This however, was to be kept separate from the daily attendance book used by other staff.

Professionally things were going well in 1868. The establishment at Earlswood had developed an international reputation. A request had been received from the founders of the Stewart Asylum in Dublin for their newly appointed Medical Superintendent, Dr Frederick Kidd, to spend some time at Earlswood so as to ensure that the new Dublin institution would follow the successful lines of management already established by John Langdon Down. Langdon Down had seen the total number of residents climb from 276 in 1859 to 455 in 1868. The emphasis was always on five-year admissions, with a view to early training. The average age on admission fell from 14 years in 1858 to 11 years in 1866.

Apart from dealing with an ever-increasing number of admissions, Langdon Down steered Earlswood from crisis to crisis as one epidemic after another struck the institution over the years. In 1864 a virulent form of scarlet fever affected 147 residents and 45 staff. Langdon Down reported on the epidemic in detail in the *London Hospital Reports* in 1864. He described 65 cases as simple, 78 as anginose, implying that they had a heavily infected membrane on their tonsils, and 49 cases as being malignant, indicating that they were highly toxic.

Only one of the 49 attendants died. This patient had not long recovered from acute rheumatic fever, in which he had developed cardiac complications, including inflammation of the pericardium. Langdon Down put his faith in treatment with sesquicarbonate of ammonia but, nevertheless, six of his 145 enfeebled residents died. He took pride in the low overall mortality among his patients. Other series at that time quoted a mortality as high as 10%, but the mortality in Earlswood was less than 5%[4].

There was no isolation accommodation in Earlswood so he cleared one large ward and mobilized staff from all departments of the hospital. He assigned nursing duties to seamstresses and housemaids. Miss Ruddick, an assistant school mistress, earned his special praise. In writing to the Board he drew attention to her special services, requesting a bonus for her:

> At a time when nearly the whole household were panic-stricken she brought to my aid a clear head and an untiring arm in carrying out the various measures of my suggestion. When servant after servant sickened and fell ill, she willingly responded to my call for services to which I had no claim and which independently of her inherent worth intended to improve the morale of the servant staff and have an indirect influence of great value. Early and late she was to be seen taking the lead in the sick wards, and offices which were worse than menial and such that all female delicacy, except under the stimulus of a high sense of duty would have rebelled at. I am not sure whether you would feel it right to advise the Board to make her some tangible amount in appreciation of her work. I feel, however, quite sure that I should be wanting in gratitude did I not thus prominently call your attention to the great value of her aid at a time of severe need and at the height of a great calamity[5].

The Board accepted his suggestion and Miss Ruddick's salary was increased from £25 to £30 per annum when the epidemic abated. Langdon Down reported on his experience of the treatment of scarlet fever in the *London Hospital Reports* in 1864[6]. Before the epidemic ended he had seen 192 cases. In comparing his 5% mortality to other reported experiences, he made specific reference to Dr James Miller, formerly Assistant Physician at the London Hospital who had had 21 deaths in a series of 219 patients. He made an important point with regard to the mortality, explaining that the patients who died were mainly in the imbecile class, a class he said in which resistance to disease of any kind is low, in which life expectancy is no more than one third of the normal life span and in which nursing is very difficult. He was very proud of the Earlswood mortality record; during the years 1859–65 it ranged from 0.5% admissions during non-epidemic years to 5% during epidemics.

The other two epidemic diseases which caused concern were measles and typhoid. In 1863 a severe epidemic of measles occurred, involving 120 patients and 16 deaths (13%). In 1866 a smaller epidemic of 56 cases occurred and this was reported to be a milder form of the disease. Nevertheless there were six deaths among the 52 cases (11%). Presumably it was milder only in the sense that there were fewer complications. A crude measles mortality of 11–13% is as high as might be seen today in the developing world. Bacterial complications which followed a severe course in the enfeebled disabled residents of Earlswood, led to deaths which would not now occur in the antibiotic era. Typhoid occurred in epidemic form in 1860 and five of the 15 affected patients died

(30%). Earlswood escaped cholera and diphtheria and, although there was an outbreak of cholera in nearby Reigate in 1866, no cases occurred in Earlswood. An isolation ward was badly needed but it was not until 1877 that one was opened.

In the throes of all these clinical crises his enthusiasm for observation and classification never flagged. He had written seven papers in medical journals and had a further three in preparation. His second son, Reginald, was also born during this time, in 1866. Langdon Down had turned his back on the private suggestion that he should, in 1863, accept the shared Chair of Physiology in the London Hospital Medical School. This issue arose again in 1866 and, on June 4th, the minutes of the Medical Council of the London Hospital recorded a decision that Dr Morell MacKenzie should be appointed to share the lectures with Dr Hughlings Jackson, provided that no other applications had been received by the time of the next meeting. Reading between the lines the overtures which had been made to Langdon Down in 1863 may have been made once more but, in spite of occasional differences with the Board of the Earlswood Asylum for Idiots, he was well-settled in his post. From 1865 he had the specific sanction of the Board for his attendance at the London Hospital twice weekly. His appointment in the London Hospital had, until that time, never been formally recognized in writing. The Board however, clearly wanted to make certain that this arrangement was not abused and stipulated that the times of leaving and returning to the Asylum of the Superintendent should be regularly recorded[7].

His standing with the Commissioners in Lunacy was very high. At their last inspection of Earlswood before his resignation he had the satisfaction of knowing that the only criticism expressed by them was that the residents of the lowest class in the probationary wards were still poorly supplied with toys and games and that their rooms were not attractive. The Commissioners were of the opinion that not enough was being attempted in the way of training for them[8]. The visitors also suggested that the younger boys be looked after by female rather than male attendants. This was indeed something that Langdon Down immediately arranged in his own private institution when it came to be opened. However he left Earlswood before the change could be made there.

He did not always get his own way. In December 1864 the Board had taken umbrage at the application of a Mrs Hopley for the admission of her grandson in which she had said that Dr Down had considered him to be a suitable case for admission. Dr Langdon Down was directed to instruct Mrs Hopley to remove the reference to his name from her application. In a sense, the Board was short-sighted. Their objection was based on principle. They viewed Langdon Down as an employee and the admission of patients as a matter for the Governors. They wished to make it clear that he was excluded from the inner councils of the Asylum. Unfortunately, they did not realize that good administration can make for a good institution, but that, in the medical field, only the work of great doctors can make an institution truly great. He was no longer a fledgling and it might take more than an increase in his salary to command his continuing loyalty[9].

His friend John Conolly died in 1866. In addition he was in danger of having to proceed without the support of his other good friend and supporter Dr Little. Little had given up his appointment at the London Hospital, writing that he would not abandon the duties and responsibilities of his office before the expiration of his legal tenure unless he experienced increasing difficulty, owing to the demands of private practice and the distance at which he now resided. Abandoning the unpaid work of a hospital in face of increased commitment to private practice was not unusual, although Langdon Down never followed this course. He was exemplary in continuing with his voluntary hospital work until the end of the appointed term.

Langdon Down was a teacher and considered it important for medical students to have some instruction on learning difficulties. He wanted to bring them from the London Hospital for hands-on experience in the Earlswood Asylum. A special committee, set up in 1863 had failed to proceed on the matter[10]. This was a committee of the Board, which Dr Down was to attend. The motion had been proposed by Mr Gunnell but when the proposer did not present himself at the special meeting, the motion to accept the students and to provide a special course of lectures for them was deemed under bye-law to have been withdrawn. The matter was never raised again.

Another matter which must have disappointed Langdon Down was the refusal to allow the world-famous Dr Séguin, formerly of Paris and then of New York, to visit Earlswood as part of his preparation for a new edition of his book. He had written in 1863 to ask if he might travel from New York to spend a few months with Langdon Down[11]. The question was referred for reply to Dr Conolly and Dr Séguin's request was turned down. It is difficult to understand why. It is possible that the Governors were of the opinion that in the Asylum they were the proprietors of a patented system which they wished to monopolize. The Board may also have been concerned at the cost implications and reluctant to increase their funding for the medical department, even although it would have been for a matter of three months only. It may also have been viewed as an inappropriate use of charity funds, without immediate or direct benefit to the patients. Conolly's health was failing and he may not have fully realized the advantages which might accrue from Séguin's visit. The request from the Stewart Hospital, already mentioned, was acceded to only after persistent application.

Séguin and Down were probably the two clearest thinkers in the field of provision for the learning disabled. A period of close association could clearly have advanced medical knowledge a great deal but this was not to be, although Langdon Down and Séguin became good friends by correspondence and held each other in high regard. In 1887, when Dr G Harley FRS proposed Langdon Down's toast at Normansfield, he spoke of a letter he had received from Séguin about an impending visit to London in which Séguin had written: 'I would not leave London without meeting the man who has done the most for idiots in England'[12].

These were relatively minor setbacks. Langdon Down had a sense of equanimity and did not allow these minor irritations to provoke any reaction on his part. Within Earlswood he showed great enthusiasm for the workshops and the handicrafts produced there. Earlswood dealt mainly with residents who had come from lower middle class backgrounds. The hope that they would acquire some vocational skills and become employable was of great importance; the handicrafts were not just a hobby. In 1867 a world exhibition was to be held in Paris and Langdon Down got approval for arranging an exhibit of the work of William Henry Pullen, one of the Earlswood residents. In due course the exhibit was awarded a bronze medal. An agent was paid to transport the material, to hire an exhibition case and ensure that all went well. Additionally, Langdon Down intended to be in Paris to make a presentation[13]. His intention was to be in Paris one week before and one week after the exhibition. The Board was of the opinion that the advantages likely to accrue to the Institution by the exhibition of articles sent to Paris did not justify their sanctioning the proposed absence of Dr Down or of paying expenses beyond those which they might agree to pay to the agent already engaged by Dr Down. He wrote to the Board expressing his relief at not having to travel to Paris but was clearly offended at the limits being set on his expansion plans for one of his projects. The certificate awarded at the Paris Exhibition was framed and placed in the Board Room[14].

He took a pragmatic view of paying patients, realizing that they brought both income and prestige to the Institution. In 1858 the Board had decided that at no future date should the number of payment cases exceed the election cases[15]. Applications for the election places usually numbered 150 for the 35 or so places available. Accommodation for paying patients was always limited. This policy had been rigidly enforced and, indeed, the number of paying patients was below 50%. In 1864 Langdon Down suggested that more vacancies should be reserved for paying patients and that the Board should reverse it's policy. He also suggested that payments for all categories of paying patients should be increased and pointed out that this would also provide an additional source of income[16]. He had a valid point. He based his suggestion on the evidence that the standard fee for a private patient was set at a level which barely covered the average costs incurred. Average costs at that time were approximately £46 per year and the excess income generated by a private case was only £4.

A special category of resident who paid £150–£250 per annum was established. They had single room accommodation and an individually assigned attendant. They were also allowed to dine in a separate dining room. These special patients were admitted and were known as parlour patients. Some paying patients had their fees abated and paid no more than £25 per annum[17]. The Board was divided in its opinion on this matter. One of those who supported the idea of increasing the benefits accruing from the accommodation of private patients was William Banting. Banting was a well-known benefactor of private institutions and famous in his own right for having, although only a layman, promoted a successful weight-loss diet. Langdon Down was later to use the diet to good effect in some of his obese patients.

There was an unsatisfied demand for accommodation for upper-class patients but the Board was resistant to the idea of increasing their numbers. One member of the Board went so far as to say that the founding father, the Reverend Andrew Reed, had only accepted the admission of upper-class patients as a temporary expedient and that the real intention of the institution was that it should function as a charity. The borderline patients whose fees were abated from £50 were clearly being subsidized. Likewise, life payment cases admitted on the basis of a single payment of £500 were something of a time-bomb. When Langdon Down left Earlswood there were over 150 of these. Their acceptance, however, relieved parental anxiety concerning long-term care and from 1865 onwards, one life case was accepted for every five charity patients elected.

Election cases were accepted on fixed election dates in April and November. Payment cases could be admitted at any time. Votes in the election of a patient were based on the value of subscriptions registered on behalf of the proposers. An annual subscription of one guinea entitled the subscriber to two votes. A one off compounded subscription of £10 conveyed the same privilege. Elections took place between 12 noon and 2 pm at the London Tavern in Bishopsgate Street. A postal vote could be cast. The voting paper gave the candidate's name, age, address, occupation of father or mother, dependent siblings and which of the parents were alive. Votes could be carried over from one election to another.

The Langdon Downs went outside the limits of the Earlswood system and, without prior approval of the Board, set up an outreach programme. A number of patients were placed in the homes of staff members and other local families, to be supervised by Mary Langdon Down. The non-resident patients may perhaps have used the Earlswood school. Miss Fagg, the school headmistress, always referred in her reports to day pupils and night pupils. Langdon Down was debarred from off-site activity of this kind, but his wife, Mary, was not a hospital employee.

The Langdon Downs' independent service might never have come to light were it not for a letter written by an anxious mother to the secretary of the Board enquiring about the condition of her son. The secretary wrote back to say that no such individual was under the care of the institution but the mother wrote again to explain that her child was not resident in the institution but was under the care of the Medical Superintendent, Dr Down. The Board instituted an enquiry[18]. The house committee also convened an enquiry in January, 1868. Langdon Down was requested to report further but he later declined to answer the questions of the Board[19]. The Board took issue with the unapproved arrangements. Before the Board enquiry could take place Langdon Down tendered his resignation.

Langdon Down wrote to the Board pointing out that four patients had been accommodated by two employees. He distanced himself from personal involvement in the supervision and education of the patients concerned. The wife of Everett had formerly taken in needlework and the wife of Walker had formerly kept a small draper's shop[20]. Between them they had four patients, placed by their relatives under Mrs Down's care and surveillance. These were patients who had been unable to secure admission to the Asylum and were awaiting vacancies. He added that there were other patients in the houses of persons quite unconnected with the Asylum who were also under Mrs Down's care and daily superintendence. Families in each case fully knew that she alone was responsible. He had no hesitation in sanctioning such arrangements. While meeting for a time the pressing needs of the clients of the Asylum, it also conserved the interests of the Institution by preserving desirable patients for forthcoming vacancies who would otherwise have been lost.

> Moreover, I held the opinion, which I still entertain, that Mrs Down, Mrs Everett and Mrs Walker, so long as what they did was not conflicting with the interests of the Asylum but was preservative thereof, were free to add to the incomes of their husbands by this means, as Mrs Down would be to engage in literature, Mrs Walker to keep shop, Mrs Everett to take in dressmaking or Mrs Wood, the schoolmaster's wife who is charge of nine children[20].

It was agreed to convene a special sub-committee but Langdon Down must have had forewarning of the expected outcome and, when they met on 10 February, he had tabled a further letter which read:

Gentlemen,

After due consideration of the reasons which have become cumulative I beg to resign the trust with which you have honoured me... Although dissevered I shall feel an interest in the continued success of the charity with which some of my best years have been associated.

Wishing you every prosperity in the work of which you have the management,

I am, gentlemen,

> Your obedient servant

> J Langdon Down[21]

Langdon Down may have been concerned that other matters relating to his contract were likely to be reviewed. He lodged with the Board a payment of 10 guineas which had been made to him by the family of a patient. He was, of course, not entitled to receive fees and he may have been pressed by the family to accept the gift for special services. The Board did not institute any specific enquiry into this rather delicate matter. He also handed in a payment for £4.12s.10d for bazaar goods sold and 13s.6d collected by 'a lady'. Presumably the lady was his wife Mary.

The Committee considered the letter and it was unanimously agreed that his resignation be accepted, assuring him at the same time that he was quite in error in assuming that the Committee had come to foregone conclusions in relation to this matter. The Committee met with Langdon Down on 25 March. He was asked to say at what time he could conveniently leave. He promised to consider the subject and write to the Board and replied naming 15 April as his departure date. And so he left Earlswood. Frederick Everett also saw the writing on the wall. He left before he could be dismissed but was not to be unemployed for long and shortly began a personal association with Langdon Down which was to last for over 30 years. When Langdon Down developed the Normansfield, Frederick Everett emerged again as an attendant and his name is inscribed on a commemorative plaque in the Normansfield theatre. In 1879 he was the recipient of a special presentation following completion of 21 years service.

There was trouble ahead. On 3 June it was reported that Langdon Down, with two gentlemen, had gone over the asylum unaccompanied by any officer. The committee decreed that Dr Down should not be allowed to enter the asylum again without permission. Dr Westall was appointed locum and enquired of the house committee concerning a book containing the history of cases that were and had been in the asylum. This could not be found[22]. Dr

Westall had no doubt that such a book existed because he had done locum work there in the past.

The Board was of the opinion that such a record had been kept and wrote to Dr Down if he would be good enough to forward this book to the Board at his earliest convenience. On 17 June a reply arrived from Langdon Down stating he had no such book as the one asked for by the Board. The matter was referred to by the Visitors[23]. They recorded that it was their duty to direct attention to the fact that 159 leaves had been cut from the casebooks relating to the progress and treatment of as many patients who had either left the Asylum or died therein. The various statements relating to these patients on admission still remained, the only addition being the part of their death or discharge, the date of either being in most instances omitted plus, in addition, the cause of death.

The Visitors noted that the Commissioners in Lunacy had failed to ascertain or discover the author of this grave offence. The finger was pointed at Langdon Down. He wrote again on 17 July, 1868 to say that he was not in the possession of the book. The Normansfield records in the London Metropolitan Records Office (LMRO) appear to confirm his position. The registers of admissions to Normansfield compiled by Langdon Down, which included the names and dates of admission of his earlier patients to the Royal Earlswood Asylum, are so incomplete in relation to the Earlswood data that he clearly could not have had immediately available to him retrospective data from Earlswood that would have enabled him to fill gaps in his series[24]. A review of the Earlswood records confirms that the statutory patients casebooks, male and female, are intact. The other statutory requirement was that a book should be kept with an entry for each patient giving all the relevant personal details and with additional columns for the outcome, either discharge or death. Scrutiny of this admission register confirms that the first 159 pages covering the admissions to 1858 have been removed. The facts are incontrovertible. Langdon Down clearly left Earlswood unexpectedly and at short notice. He was involved in an ongoing study of his case material. It is possible, but unlikely, that in a panic reaction, and fearing for the loss of continuity in his records he did, indeed, extract the pages concerned. The clinical observations could be viewed as being, in part at least, his intellectual property. The evidence however, is against his having been the mutilator of the records.

Looking at the numbered photographs which Langdon Down took of his patients, it is clear that they are arranged in a numerical sequence which does not correspond to the register of admissions in the LMRO, nor does it correspond to the numerical reference numbers of male and female patients in the official casebooks in the Surrey Records Office. He clearly kept a personal register with a different numbering system which he took with him when he left Earlswood, but unfortunately this has not survived, making it difficult to match the clinical records and the associated mid-century photographs. He had referred in public so frequently to his notebooks that there clearly was widespread appreciation of the fact that he had compiled them. They were, however, his personal intellectual property and indeed formed the basis for his publications. Dr Westall had probably seen Langdon Down's notebooks in the Medical Superintendent's office. These were not, however, the hospital records but Langdon Down's personal records. The affair remains clouded in mystery.

The Commissioners in Lunacy, having looked into the matter, failed to reach any conclusion concerning the missing entries which had been extracted from the record books and the matter was dropped. Dr Grabham, Langdon Down's successor as Medical Superintendent, made an ongoing complaint about a patient called Eborall, concerning whom he had been unable to trace any note of any kind in the general register of patients, and about another patient called Westoff, who had had no note made from the time of his admission in July 1858. On 4 November 1868, a letter from Langdon Down was tabled, saying that the patient Westoff was working on the farm in 1858 and was still there in 1868, unchanged[25]. The patient Eborall had probably arrived late in the evening without accompanying relatives and in an excited state. His admission note was, in consequence, postponed and subsequently overlooked. Langdon Down confirmed that he had not, nor had he authorized, the removal of any notes. This carefully phrased reply may, however, not exclude the possibility that a member of staff, angered by the circumstances in which Langdon Down was leaving Earlswood, decided to remove the accumulated record of his work and give it to him. Langdon Down was very highly regarded by the staff and they, independently of the Board, made a presentation to him when he left. His well-balanced reply, saying that he had not himself removed the pages, nor had he authorized the removal, would still allow of the possibility that a well-meaning clerical assistant may have removed the pages on Langdon Down's behalf. In the circumstances it would have been very difficult to return them if they had come into his possession.

Langdon Down had served Earlswood well. From 1858 to 1865 he had worked single-handed. It was seven years before an assistant medical officer was appointed. Distinguished medical visitors from Switzerland, Sweden, Holland and the US travelled to see the workings of an institution which had become a centre of excellence. Writing in 1869 Dr James Clark of the London Hospital, by now a Knight Commander of the Bath and Physician in Ordinary to the Queen, wrote of Langdon Down:

> His retirement is a great public loss. He filled his position in the Earlswood asylum in a way in which no man has filled a similar

position in this country or in any country in Europe. I give this, not as my own opinion, but I believe it to be the general opinion among those who are giving attention to imbecile children. Dr Down was a scientific man, and he greatly advanced our knowledge of idiocy, and what he did gave promise of much more. He was an earnest, able, working man, such as it was most desirable to see at the head of our greatest institution, and in the direction of public opinion on this subject[26].

Soured relationships were never restored. Langdon Down's successor proceeded to report in later years on the progress of the Asylum in terms which almost indicated that Langdon Down had never existed and no word of thanks ever came down from the Board. This must have been a time of great crisis. His wife Mary was expecting her third son, Percival. The question of accommodation for patients in the upper income group had exercised his mind and Langdon Down had previously acquired site plans of available property in Redhill, possibly with the idea of building an auxiliary institution for the upper classes. He had also quickly assessed the possibility of a private building development in Wimbledon. He wrote a letter to his contacts setting out his position:

> I beg to inform you that I have resigned the position I have held for nearly 10 years of Medical Superintendent of the asylum at Earlswood and propose establishing a private institution for the care and training of the feeble minded and backward among the higher classes. I have secured desirable premises and grounds in a healthy site near Wimbledon Common where I hope to be able to offer superior advantages. I shall be assisted in the management by Mrs Down, who has for eight years largely aided me in directing the training of the female division at Earlswood. As the Board of Management of Earlswood have advertised that they are not prepared to receive further applications from payment cases, may I ask you to mention my plans to any persons having afflicted children to whom the information may be useful[27].

His plans changed, and instead of moving to Wimbledon he moved to Normansfield in Hampton Wick, near Teddington.

Langdon Down's resignation has been viewed unsympathetically by Dr Wright, who has analysed the event as simply a move towards financial advancements quoting his salary on leaving as £500. It was, in fact, £700 (£42,000 today), and the financial loss, especially taking into account the free lodgings, was considerable[28]. In moving to develop a service for private patients Mary and John Langdon Down were sailing in uncharted waters and undertaking a major capital investment with no guarantee of success and haunted by the family folk-memory of the effects of bankruptcy. That they did in fact succeed was a great credit to both of them.

References

1. Surrey Record Office. SRO;392/2/1/4. Board Minutes, March 11th, 1863.
2. Royal London Hospital Minutes of the Association Lecturers. 17 December, 1862.
3. Surrey Record Office. SRO;392/2/1/5. Board Minutes, F181.
4. Down JLD. Treatment of scarlet fever by the sesquicarbonate of ammonia. *London Hospital Reports* 1864; **1**: 159–61.
5. Surrey Record Office. SRO;392/1/2/1. Annual Report, F259.
6. *London Hospital Reports* 1864; **1**: 159–61.
7. Surrey Record Office. SRO;392/2/1/5. Board Minutes, F205.
8. Surrey Record Office. SRO;392/10/1/1. Visitor's Report. 17 November, 1868.
9. Surrey Record Office. SRO;392/2/1/5. Board Minutes, F161.
10. Surrey Record Office. SRO;392/2/1/4. Board Minutes, F421.
11. Surrey Record Office. SRO;392/2/1/5. Board Minutes, F8.
12. Surrey Comet. 9th July, 1987.
13. Surrey Record Office. SRO;392/2/1/6.F17.
14. Surrey Record Office. SRO;392/1/2/1. Annual report. F365.
15. Surrey Record Office. SRO;392/2/2/2. Board Minutes. April 28th, 1858.
16. Surrey Record Office. SRO;392/2/8/1. Letters. June 4th, 1864.
17. Surrey Record Office. SRO;392/1/2/1. Matters Arising, House Committee: 25–9.
18. Surrey Record Office. SRO;392/2/5: 25–7.
19. Surrey Record Office. SRO;392/3/1/10. House Committee, F250.
20. Surrey Record Office. SRO;392/3/1/11. House Committee, F131.
21. Surrey Record Office. SRO;392/3/1/11. House Committee, F137.
22. Surrey Record Office. SRO;392/3/1/11. House Committee, F183.
23. Surrey Record Office. SRO;392/10/1/1. House Committee, F17.
24. London Metropolitan Records Office. LMRO;829/NF/B/1/1.
25. Surrey Record Office. SRO;392/2/1/6. House Committee, F247.
26. Clark J. *Memoir of John Conolly*. John Murray, 1869.
27. Unpublished correspondence.
28. Wright D. *The National Asylum for Idiots, Earlswood. 1847–1886*. Unpublished PhD Thesis. University of Oxford, 1993.

Chapter 9

Normansfield

When the Langdon Downs moved into Normansfield in 1868 John Langdon Down was 40 years old. Mary was 39 and in the final stages of her fourth pregnancy; Percival was born within a week of them going to live there. The decision to buy Normansfield must have been taken very quickly. It was a large white gentleman's residence developed along with two others. Five acres of ground went with the house. A fourth residence planned for the site was never developed. In due course, Langdon Down acquired the other two houses and land. The purchase price of the house was £3,388 and furniture and books cost £612, making a total of £4,000. The Langdon Downs had not had any great opportunity to acquire capital. Personal family accounts show that, between them, husband and wife had approximately £4000 in savings, probably including Mary's dowry[1].

When they bought the house it was called the White House. They changed the name to Normansfield. It was common knowledge that the change was made in tribute to Mr Norman Wilkinson, senior partner in a law firm in Brockley and a friend of Langdon Down. The money for the first purchase was raised by a mortgage and the likelihood is that Norman Wilkinson, through his legal contacts, identified a willing investor. A mortgage of £4,300 was arranged[2]. The security for the mortgage was the Normansfield lease. When the other properties were acquired Langdon Down took out further mortgages. Ultimately, the total mortgages amounted to £43,591, approximately one-quarter of which had been contributed through Mary Langdon Down's family and relatives. The increased financial backing ultimately resulted in the total acreage of the property increasing to over 40 acres, and extending from Normansfield Road to Holmesdale Road and from Kingston Road to Broom Road, with a tongue of land extending towards the river-bank.

The Langdon Downs had to face two further problems. Now cut off from salaried employment, John Langdon Down had to make a start in developing a consulting practice. To do this he had to face ongoing outlay over the period of time it took to first balance his practice costs and then move into a credit situation. He began by renting consulting rooms at 39 Welbeck Street, an address at which he continued to practise for the next 13 years. In order to be more clearly identifiable, he changed his name to Langdon-

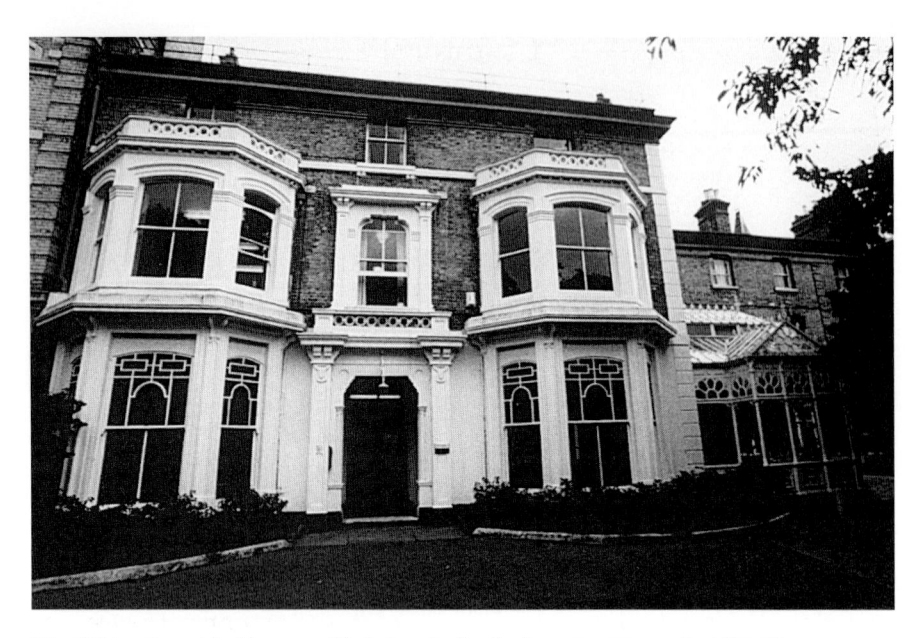

The 'White House' in Hampton Wick, bought by the Langdon Downs in 1868. The name was changed to Normansfield.

Down. He had always used Langdon as his forename, signing his earliest letters J Langdon H Down. The decision to choose this identification of a line of descent was not motivated by the intention to make false claims to distinguished ancestry. If he had wanted to do this he could have chosen the Haydon connection with greater justification as this had a stronger claim to notable forbears. From here on he was John Langdon Haydon Langdon-Down. As a matter of interest, 'Langdon-Down' sometimes appears hyphenated and sometimes not; it is hyphenated on his commemorative stone in Normansfield, but not in his 1887 Will signature, or in the 1881 census. All the descendants of John Langdon Down used the hyphenated surname 'Langdon-Down'. However, for the sake of simplicity and consistency, the name 'Langdon Down' is used throughout this book.

Langdon Down made the journey in and out of London to Welbeck Street and the London Hospital in his coach. This round trip had to be made on a regular basis until 1881 when he purchased 81 Harley Street. He carried on his practice at the new address from then on and, being the owner of the whole house, could stay there overnight if necessary, if his workload required it, or if he had a late night social engagement. His coachman, Walter Lee, was long-serving and was among the first employees to receive an award for 21 years' service.

In the first year at Normansfield, 19 patients were admitted. The census for subsequent years was as follows[3]:

Year	Number of patients	Year	Number of Patients
1869	22	1883	137
1870	30	1884	149
1871	37	1885	143
1872	49	1886	139
1873	57	1887	135
1874	75	1888	135
1875	90	1889	147
1876	95	1890	146
1877	100	1891	143
1878	106	1892	152
1879	117	1893	154
1880	117	1894	156
1881	129	1895	154
1882	145	1896	145

The purchase of the two adjoining properties increased the potential capacity of the institution. They were used in the main for individuals with mild learning difficulties. From 1882 the additional patients in the satellite units in Eastcote (renamed Trematon) and Conifers increased the overall total by 30 to 40 and, in 1896 when John Langdon Down died, the number of residents under his care was 181. The annual increase in the number of patients was halted in 1886. This was a year when many people suffered losses in stocks and shares and so there was reduced spending among the upper classes.

Initially major expansion had to take place rapidly. The south wing was added in 1869 and in 1872 the foundation stone of the north wing was laid. This was completed by the end of 1873. For each extension a commemorative plaque was commissioned. Everleigh, the eldest son, was commemorated in this way in 1873, Reginald in 1877 and Percival in 1878. The Langdon Down family lived in and for Normansfield and the two generations, later followed by a third, were meshed in its development. When the expansion programme was complete the total mortgages of the Langdon Downs were the equivalent of £2.25 million in today's terms. This represented a very courageous programme for a man whose youth had been lived under the shadow of his father's earlier bankruptcy. The remaining mortgage was paid off in 1893 and was a cause for celebration; the Langdon Downs were free of debt. Their two sons were in medical school, Reginald in his first post as a house physician to the famous Hughlings Jackson and Percival in his final year at the London Hospital.

In a public gesture of affirmation of their belief that man's life was in the hands of a Creator who could bless or mar it, the Langdon

Downs commissioned a mosaic inset in the wall of the stairwell of the entrance to the Normansfield theatre which had been opened in 1879 (see chapter 12). They had been blessed and wished to acknowledge it. The mosaic depicts the Divine Creator holding the orb of the world in his hand, with the inscription; 'Blessing and honour and glory and power be unto him that sitteth upon the throne[4]'. The mosaic is in a way sad. In each corner there is an angel. Two of the angels are in a

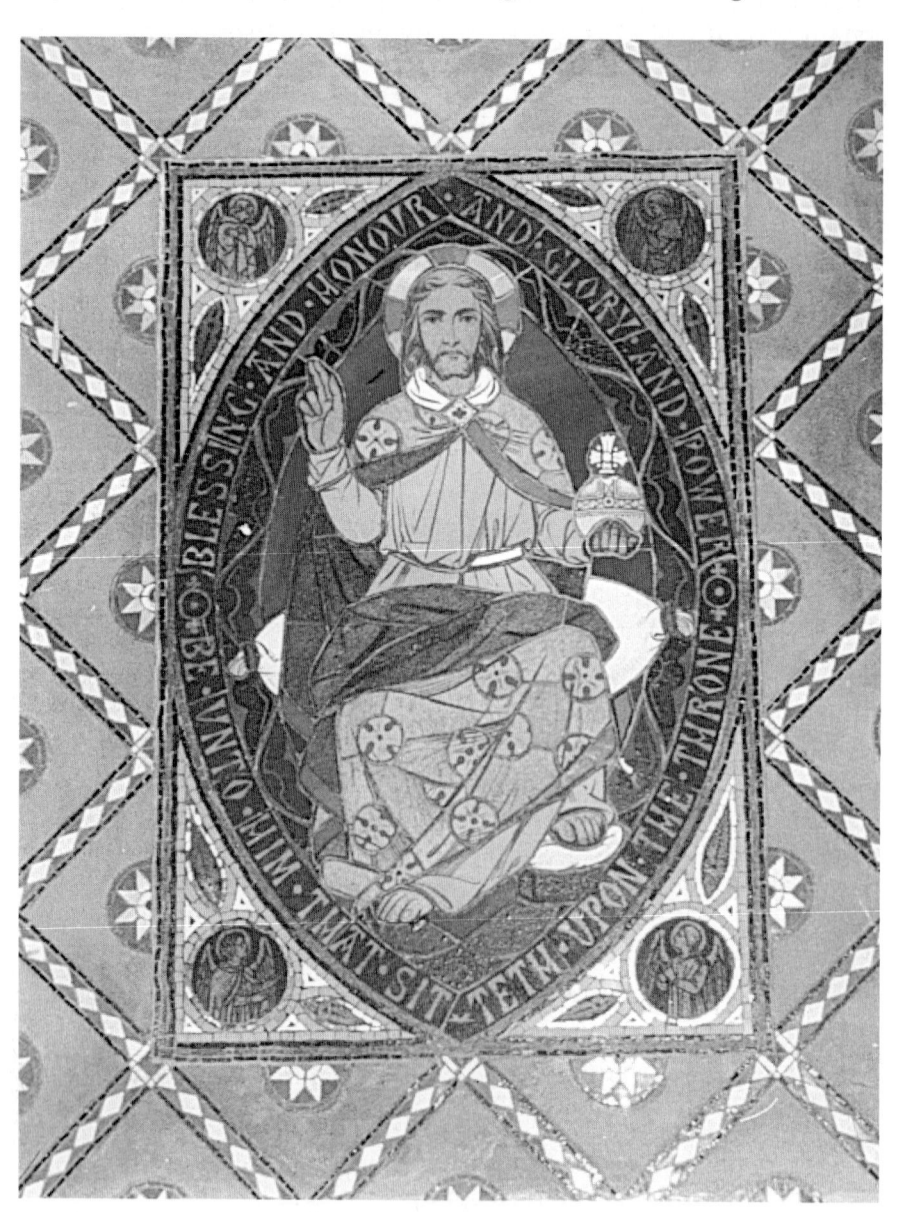

The Rush mosaic, commissioned in 1893. The inscription reads: 'Blessing and honour and glory be unto him that sitteth upon the throne'. The Langdon Downs were devout Christians.

position of repose with arms folded across their chests. Two walk with arms outstretched and it is tempting to speculate that the angels in repose represent a memorial to the son and daughter whose lives were prematurely cut short.

The adjacent properties were purchased between 1875 and 1882 and, in 1873, the strip of land running down to the river was purchased; it was here in 1884 that the boathouse was built. The sons Reginald and Percival were now in their twenties and, when the opportunity arose, they became enthusiastic sailors. They sailed a one and half ton sloop called *Cats Eye* and the family became prominently connected with the Tamesis Sailing Club. Then, as now, owning a boat was like owning a hole in the water into which money disappeared. The family papers include bills for a new mahogany thwart, damage to a transom and staining and making good paintwork. Rowing boats were frequently hired from Turk and Son, presumably for patients. Rowing became a family tradition and Reginald and Percival excelled at this sport at Cambridge. The family bought their first river gig in 1882 and a second in 1885. The latter was clearly very superior and their favourite niece, Miss Raines, wrote; 'it is sure to be as good as a gig can be... you must have greatly enjoyed your marine residence and the boating this year'[5]. Reginald and Percival bought plans for a sailing canoe and painstakingly built it in the Normansfield workshops. They were

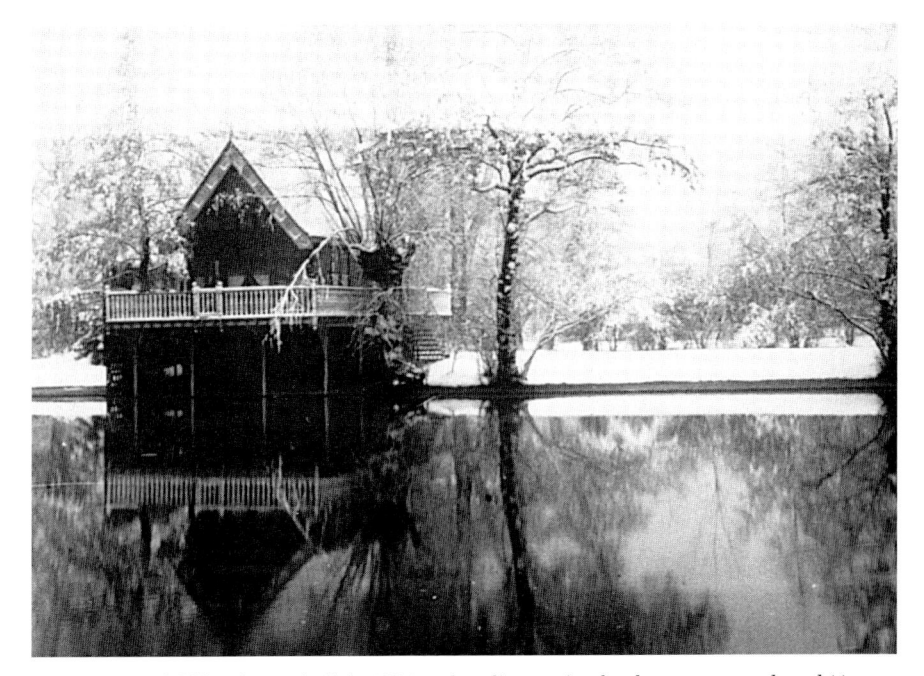

The Normansfield boathouse, built in 1884 on the adjacent riverbank property purchased 11 years previously. The date of the photograph may be 1886, when the snowfall was so heavy that Normansfield had to purchase a snowplough.

enthusiastic, if not particularly successful, sailors, despite their rowing experience.

The First Admissions

The home was registered in the name of Mrs Down. In theory at least, John Langdon Down was the Medical Superintendent. This situation persisted until 1894 when husband and wife entered into a partnership agreement, at the time their last remaining mortgages for their extensive property purchases had been paid off. The first patient to be admitted was a 21-year-old, William C, with cerebral palsy, coincidentally of the type initially described by Langdon Down's friend and mentor, Dr Little. The condition was ascribed to the effects of sunstroke, a hazard of the long journey from India via the Suez Canal. In severe sunstroke the combination of excessively high temperature and the loss of salt and water from sweating has the potential to cause convulsions. In William C's case the severity of the convulsions caused brain damage. William C had been a patient in Earlswood; he was one of the many patients who followed Langdon Down to Normansfield and lived there until he died, 20 years later, of pneumonia. All but one of the next five patients had also been taken out of Earlswood to continue under the care of Langdon Down. Christopher N, aged 9 years, suffered from athetoid cerebral palsy. He had irregular movements which made feeding difficult and he was spoon-fed by the staff. He lived to the age of 36, having had a troublesome cough and diarrhoea. He may have had cystic fibrosis and he died of bronchitis. Mary A was the first case of Down's syndrome to be admitted.

There was one other case of Down's syndrome, Herbert H, who came in as a baby aged eight months. Charles C was 31 years of age on admission and suffered from epilepsy. His fits were controlled with bromide. He died at the age of 56 from cerebral haemorrhage. Charles S was the third patient to be admitted on the opening day. He suffered from uncomplicated learning disability and lived to the age of 38. Arthur H was admitted at the age of 17 years. Although his heart was normal on admission, at the age of 28 he developed signs of progressive cardiac failure. There was no clear history of rheumatic fever but he had developed a cardiac murmur and cardiac enlargement, suggesting that he had indeed had rheumatic fever and that his heart was affected, but without sufficient joint involvement to have attracted attention. Non-articular rheumatic fever has a tendency to run an unfavourable course. When patients develop rheumatic fever with arthritis their discomfort brings them quickly to medical care. In the absence of arthritis, progressive heart disease may develop insidiously and, because precautions are not taken in time, the outcome is poor.

Of the patients admitted in the first year, seven were to die later of pneumonia. The availability of antibiotics is the main factor that has now influenced the longer survival of those with learning disabilities. Whereas a quarter of the deaths in Earlswood were due to tuberculosis, only one of the 13 deaths among the Normansfield patients admitted in the first year was due to this. One factor in this discrepancy may have been the difference in accommodation, especially sleeping accommodation. Whereas in Earlswood the residents slept in large dormitories, in Normansfield they were in groups of three or four and the opportunities for person-to-person spread of infectious diseases were greatly reduced. One patient died two from scarlet fever two years after being admitted. Overall Normansfield was spared the experience of the death-dealing epidemics which had plagued Earlswood.

Ten of the 19 admissions in the first year had followed Langdon Down from Earlswood. The series overall confirms that the families of upper-class patients in Earlswood, who were paying substantial fees, were not fully satisfied with the accommodation and the amenities there. Twenty patients were admitted to Normansfield in 1868–9. However, Normansfield was a new unit and was as yet not well-equipped; landscape gardening had still to be done and staff remained to be recruited. There were six adults to be catered for but most of the patients were children and there were eight residents between five and 10 years of age. The families' decision to move them to Normansfield was, in its own way, a vote of confidence and trust in John Langdon Down and his wife Mary. There was nothing tangible on offer by way of inducement to them.

For the Langdon Downs, the early recruitment of a small body of patients must have been some relief in face of the financial situation in which they now found themselves. It would take time to develop a significant income from the private practice in Welbeck Street and, in the meantime, the overheads would have to be met. Work in the London Hospital was voluntary and, unlike today, members of staff received neither salary, retainer nor honorarium – apart from some fees for teaching in the medical school. The immediate omens were good as far as Normansfield was concerned; even with the limited number of admissions a profit of £1000 was made in the first year which was lodged to the capital sinking fund.

Normansfield was established essentially as an institution for the learning disabled of the upper-classes. The moves that were made to establish a special centre for these children did not, however, imply that Langdon Down was unaware of the needs of the poor. Langdon Down gave an address to the Social Science Congress in 1867, which was reprinted under the title *The Education and Training of the Feeble in Mind*[7]. The address illustrates the basis of much of

Patients Admitted 1868[6]:

Name	Age	Date	Diagnosis	Outcome
Walter JC	21	11.5.68	Spastic diplegia	Died 1888 of pneumonia
Charles S	10	11.5.68	Learning disability	Discharged improved
Charles FN	9	11.5.68	Athetoid cerebral palsy	Died 1895 of bronchitis (query cystic fibrosis)
Mary A	19	12.5.68	Down's syndrome	Died 1907 of cardiac failure
Cramer RC	31	20.5.68	Epileptic	Died 1893 of cerebral haemorrhage and hemiplegia
Alfred H	17	20.5.68	Epileptic	Died 1879 of cardiac failure, possibly post-traumatic
Thomas CM	39	23.5.68	Multiple malformations, learning disability	Died 1874 of bronchitis
Maud EA	15	2.6.68	Severe learning disability	Died 1931 of tuberculosis
Mildred EP	8	8.6.68	Cerebral palsy (athetoid)	Discharged 1871, improved; occasional seizures continued
Robert Y	5	11.6.68	Learning disability	Discharged 1870, improved
Alice LB	6	11.6.68	Epilepsy	Discharged 1873, improved
Catherine C	8	15.6.68	Severe learning disability	Died 1875 of pneumonia
Lucia AH	10	17.6.68	Athetoid cerebral palsy Foetal alcohol syndrome	Died 1879 of pneumonia
Ada MW	5	11.6.68	Learning disability	Died 1879 of severe nephritis
John TB	22	17.6.68	Mild learning disability, acute depression	Died 1907 of pneumonia
Cecelia GA	10	4.7.68	Down's syndrome	Died 1870 of scarlet fever
Claude GP	8	22.10.68	Fusion of cranial sutures, severe learning disability	Died 1879 of pneumonia
Herbert HH	8	18.7.68	Down's syndrome	Discharged September 1868, improved
William WE	14	29.7.68	Severe learning disability	Discharged 1874, not improved
Emily MW	17	6.8.68	Defect in posterior cranium. Moderate learning disability	Discharged 1876, improved

This table is based on the Normansfield Casebooks, but has been interpreted and updated by the author to be of relevance to modern readers.

Langdon Down's social thinking and is of great value in understanding the man who was its author.

The Education and Training of the Feeble in Mind

In the address Langdon makes a plea for the development of special services for the learning disabled of all classes. Affected children of poor parents were often inappropriately placed in lunatic asylums and he knew that this was not where they ought to be. He felt that charities similar to Earlswood could cater for the children of working-class parents and moved himself to provide for children of the upper classes in Normansfield. He emphasized that the problem was most common among the poor, where parents could cope least well with the special difficulties of a mentally handicapped child. For all classes, however, he identified in particular the feeling of isolation which derives from lack of accomplishment and, in striving to provide companionship within a peer group, he was led towards the institutional model of care. What he wanted to see was children of similar abilities grouped together, so as to enjoy each others' company and stimulate in each other a desire to progress.

> Probably nothing indicates more fully the onward progress of civilisation than the thought that is now being given to the waifs and strays of humanity... In a barbaric age the extermination of those who had not helped the State, or tried, was considered the wisest political economy. Even so short a period as 50 years ago, it would have been regarded as vain enthusiasm to expend care or thought on members of the community who were treated in every way as the solitary ones as their name suggests.
>
> We live, however, in times when it is not thought unsuitable at a Congress of those who are interested in the social progress of our land, to discuss the best plan for elevating and improving individuals, who without fault of their own are powerless to rescue themselves from a condition than which humanity knows nothing more pitiable, and which as yet society has made only partial efforts to relieve...
>
> The large proportion of idiocy is to be found among the lower orders, where the parents are making a desperate struggle for existence – where the afflicted child is not only a consuming member, but an incubus, paralysing the efforts of the productive, and absorbing the time and energy of at least one sane life. Ascending a step higher in the social scale, do the arrangements of middle class life meet the requirements of one who demands more than the usual appliances, to fan into a flame the flickering spark? The children of this class are either educated at school or taught at home. The imbecile cannot advantageously accompany its brothers and sisters to school, for its presence there would be

prejudicial to the establishment, even if the teaching were suited to its needs. Nor is it found that home instruction with others is more practicable. The teacher soon devotes the greatest attention to those who best repay the effort, while the feeble one falls hopelessly behind, without the benefit of individual skill, or the helpfulness of collective emulation...

Nor is his position more desirable in the houses of the wealthy. His claims are lost sight of, and the great aim is to keep his existence a secret, while no kind of companionship is established between him and the other members of the household. Moreover, the claims of society, the presence of visitors, the changes of residence, and like occurrences, tend to... lead to his being consigned to the care of servants in the upper and less frequented portions of the house, where his life must necessarily be monotonous and uninteresting[7].

He made a case for a medical model of management, although the case was not convincing. He quoted the need to improve diet, based on his observation that the brain tissue is often unduly pale, suggesting that the nutrition of its constituent nerve elements is impaired, an impression that would no longer be accepted today, although clearly an improved diet would would be of general benefit.

Other advice, such as his observation that the learning disabled need a gravel soil would now be treated with scepticism. This belief derived from his recognition that there was a lower incidence of tuberculosis in Normansfield, which was on a gravel soil, than he had seen in Earlswood, which was on a clay soil. The fact that tuberculosis was an infectious disease was not then known. He set out his views on how to manage the mentally disabled in order that their lives should be as productive, comfortable and stimulating as possible. In this paper he also mentions the condition that would later be referred to as 'Down's syndrome':

The first thing, therefore, to be done is to rescue the feeble one from this solitary life to give him the companionship of his peers, to place him in a condition where all the machinery shall move for his benefit and where he shall be surrounded by influences both of art and nature, calculated to make his life joyous, to arouse his observation, and to quicken his power of thought.

Nothing has been more clearly shown by the experience of the past and that the improvement of the imbecile can only be satisfactorily accomplished by having reference to a judicious combination of medical, physical, moral and intellectual treatment... The basis of all treatment should be medical. I mean by this that it should be founded on the principles of medicine in an enlarged sense; that it should have reference to what is known of the laws of Hygiene, Physiology, Chemistry and of Therapeutics.

Success can only be attained by keeping the patient in the highest possible health...

Many cases of imbecility, specially those which I have elsewhere described (having reference to the racial types which degeneracy imprints), as Mongolian imbeciles lose a large amount of intellectual energy in the winter, go through, in fact, a process of hibernation, their mental power being always directly as the external temperature. Moreover, the results of morbid anatomy teaches, that independently of the occasional grave defects in the cerebral mass, and the larger number of instances of want of size or of symmetry in the central nervous ganglia, there is frequently a very general deficiency of nourishment of the brain, as indicated by the pallor of the vesicular neurine. All these facts indicate that our first attention must be directed to the improvement of the nutrition of the tissues generally, and of the nervous centres in particular. This must be accomplished by the employment of a very liberal dietary... care should be taken, not only that the diet is sufficient in amount and of good quality, but that it is exhibited in a form suited to the powers of mastication of the various children.

...It is desirable that [the] residence should be on gravel soil and surrounded by well drained and well made walks in order that in our precarious climate no opportunity should be lost of daily outdoor exercise... Having placed our patient under the most favourable hygienic conditions, we enter on the special training which his circumstances demand, a work which requires the utmost enthusiasm.

Physical training must always form an important part of his education... We have to commence with the simplest movements, gradually making them more complex, and thus causing to grow up together the mandate and the result... From purposeless acts we build up a series of voluntary efforts which are applicable to the ones of daily life.

This training has to be carried out in minute detail, so that every voluntary muscle and every congerie [sic] muscle shall be called into action and trained to fulfil with rapidity the end for which they are designed. In this way the muscular system is strengthened, the various acts of prehension, locomotion and mastication are more effectually performed, the tongue becomes a willing agent, and the lips retain the saliva, the dropping of which formerly gave a repulsive characteristic to our patient...

The moral education of the imbecile is of paramount importance. While his physical and mental powers are being developed by hygienic and physiological processes, he has to be taught to subordinate his will to that of another. He has to learn obedience; that right doing is productive of pleasure and that wrong-doing is followed by the deprivation thereof... The whole staff takes its tone from the head and that tone should be one of affectionate regard for the subject in its care... The tact of the teacher will be called into exercise in devising the reward or punishment to suit the special case. It is curious how a study of the peculiarities of the patient will reveal a ready access to his moral control.

... It is even possible in some cases to raise them to an appreciation of the simple teachings of Christ, so as to influence their acts; but attempts to make them understand doctrinal tenets or sectional creeds, is, according to my experience, utterly futile... It is of the greatest importance that the teacher should ever bear in mind, that the primary object he should have, is to make the pupil self-helpful and, as far as possible, a useful working member of the community; this way more is effected for his happiness than by any other means. Mere abstract or memoriter knowledge is of little value, everything which makes him practically useful makes him proportionately happy[7].

Although his lecture was entitled 'The Education and Training of the Feeble in Mind', there is a certain lack of detail concerning the actual steps to be taken. While Duncan and Millard's 1866 book concerning Colchester Asylum set out a specific series of exercises for instruction in speaking, moving step by step through different levels, Langdon Down did not go into such great detail[8]. He was, however, more advanced than Thomas Andrew, who wrote in 1842 that idiocy could seldom be the subject of successful medical or moral treatment[9]. Down did not accept this pessimistic point of view; in his opinion, there was always scope for improvement.

At the time of Langdon Down's lecture to the Social Science Congress in 1867, the *BMJ* took its cue from the ideas that he had expressed. In an editorial on 'Idiocy and its Treatment' on 28 September, 1867 the editor refers to the 10,021 known imbeciles in England and emphasizes the lack of provision for the children of pauper families with learning disabilities. It refers, with approval, to the anticipated provision by the Irish Poor Law Commissioners, who exercised separate jurisdiction, of a charge on either the Exchequer or the rates for services for 'idiots'. The absence of suitable provision for the 'pauper idiot' was 'melancholy in the extreme'. Langdon Down's early efforts influenced the later establishment of the necessary public institutions, but it was not until the Mental Deficiency Act of 1913 that their establishment was made obligatory. Progress had already been made in the London metropolitan area and, from 1871 onwards, this gathered momentum. Darenth Training Schools hired the buildings of the London Orphan Asylum at Clacton to begin this service and, in 1876, the foundation stone of the Darenth Training School was laid[10].

In 1879 Langdon Down returned once more to a discussion of the problems of the poor. At the opening of a new wing and a theatre at Normansfield he was reported in the *Christian World*:

> The lower strata of society, for whom for the most part an election charity was a sealed avenue, and the upper classes of society for whom it was, to my mind, impossible to provide the refinement and culture which was necessary, in an institution where a life must be either isolated and therefore lacking the attention companionship alone can give or association with those whose language, habits and tastes would be a serious counterpoise to purely intellectual training. In a paper which I read at the Social Science Congress in Belfast I urged the necessity of providing in our counties, schools for the training of the feeble minded poor. Still more recently I have had the honour of working with your Lordship (the Earl of Devon), to enforce the claims of this neglected class[11].

The London Hospital

Langdon Down was well aware of the problems of the poor. His two years as resident obstetric officer in the London Hospital had brought him into the homes of the indigent and unemployed of Whitechapel and he had maintained his contact with them through his years of service as assistant physician and physician at the London Hospital.

London Hospital Address

In 1864, while he was still Assistant Physician, Langdon Down was honoured by the London Hospital with the invitation to give the introductory address at the opening of the academic year[12,13]. The address gives great insights into his ideals and the high standards which he set. He was an advocate of the recognition of patients' dignity and, before there was any question of a Patient's Charter, he recommended the steps which should be taken to maintain the quality of care. He commended the interdependence of the teaching hospital and the medical school, the former benefiting from the unpaid services of University staff, and the university benefiting from access to the clinical facilities. He cautioned students to aim high and to take the London University degree, rather than the LSA and MRCS with which he had started his career. He was embarassed by his own uncertain initial credentials.

He discussed the poor status of medical men in the army and navy. The point at issue was that they were having difficulty achieving full recognition as officers. He reminded the audience of the bravery of medical men under fire and gave, as an example, the heroic conduct of David Llewellyn, the assistant to the ship's surgeon on the

Alabama, a Confederate vessel which had wreaked havoc on Union shipping in the American Civil War, but which was ultimately sunk off Heligoland. Under fire and in the face of disaster, David Llewellyn had continued to minister to the sick and wounded and won the admiration of the English-speaking world, irrespective of their war-time sympathies[14].

Langdon Down reminded students of the sacrifices involved in a medical career but pointed out to them the importance of their caring role and the rewards which the consequent job satisfaction would bring. The human confidences they would enjoy were to be respected with unbreakable silence; their patients were to be respected and their work should be in the spirit of an Almighty God who is even-handed and just in His judgements. Langdon Down emphasized that, in the practice of medicine, their clinical experience would be as important to them as the academic curriculum. Regular hard work would be required and they should think of the sacrifices made by their families in sending them to medical school. They should exhaust their endeavours, striving for the glory of God and the benefit of man. The lecture gave a clear portrayal of a man who was, himself, full of sympathy for the hardships which he saw around him and who saw his calling as one in which he is to participate in the healing work of his Creator.

He had a highly developed social conscience. He admonished students to remember that they were dealing with sensitive spirits as well as injured bodies:

> The man with brawny hands and swarthy brow, who lies with fractured limb, is feeling, maybe for the first time in life, the abjectness of dependence and the possibility of pauperism. Let us not by word or deed intensify the poignancy of his position. In your care of fractured limb regard the broken spirit. Hark! that agonizing cry is from some poor woman, whose child, with cindered garments and charred integuments, is brought to you for aid. She would willingly sacrifice herself so intense is her love for her little one. She has to leave with you the most precious thing in her narrow world. Wound not her bleeding heart by flippant speech or rough rebuke. She has need of words of solace to calm her saddened state. That woman who comes in clothes of rusty black and wears the weeds of widowhood, could tell a tale of early happiness and affluence. She had once all that could make life lightsome. Now more eloquent than words are her attenuated form and sunken eyes. She seeks the hospital to prolong her hapless life. Speak to her kindly, for her soul is still as sensitive as when in halcyon days tears were mingled with her bridal joys. Remember that nearly all the patients who line the wards have left their homes, and cast themselves among strangers; they need some expression of sympathy to compensate

for the sacrifices they are called upon to make, and that their convalescence will often be promoted by the genial manner and kindly bearing of those who attend to their needs[12,13].

If Langdon Down had written nothing else this address would have been an important contribution to the development and maintenance of high ethical standards in the medical profession.

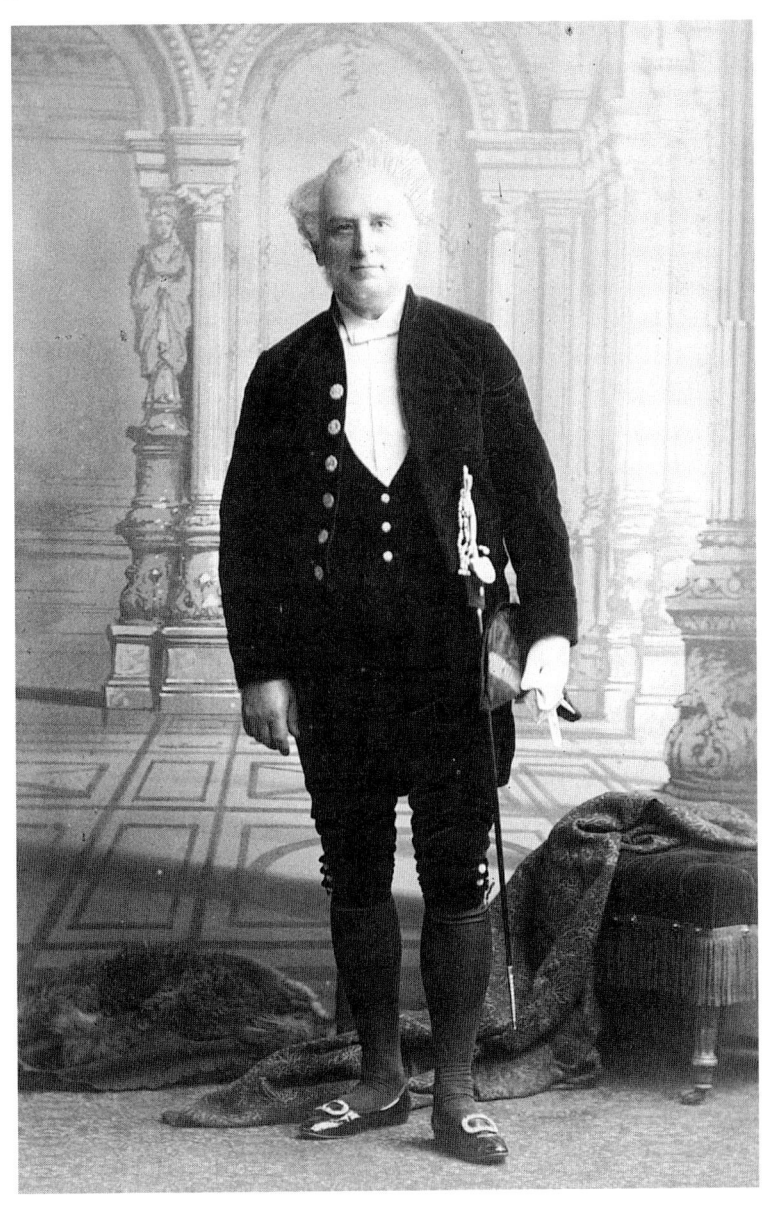

Langdon Down in court dress, 1887, when he gave the welcome address to the Prince and Princess of Wales at the opening of the London Hospital Nursing School.

At the London Hospital the question of students' fees was always an issue. Many years after the address, in 1878, there was a meeting of all the London Teaching Hospitals and, with the exception of Charing Cross, St George's and St Mary's, an increase of 25% was agreed. The Board of the London Hospital, influenced perhaps by a wish to maintain its share of student intake, decided not to join in the move for an increase in fees. Langdon Down chaired this important meeting. He was a central figure in the hospital and, when the Prince and Princess of Wales opened the nursing school in 1887, he was the hospital spokesman.

He had always been in good standing at the London Hospital and, in his earliest days as obstetric resident, the Associated Lecturers to the School of Medicine agreed that he should act as medical tutor. In 1886 he chaired many meetings of a special committee set up to consider the appointment of a medical electrician; medical science was undergoing evolution and electrical treatments for patients and radiology were becoming feasible. He was clearly a key figure in the social life of the hospital.

Local Work for the Poor

Langdon Down involved himself in other work for the poor. There was, close by in the Kingston area, a provident dispensary which was in effect a type of medical insurance club to which, through a small weekly payment, the subscribers were entitled to a medical service. Dr Coleman was the Medical Officer for the provident dispensary. John Langdon Down was not only one of the fundraisers who kept the project going, but also the honorary Medical Consultant, frequently called upon for advice. One of the biggest fundraising functions for the dispensary took place in 1891 in the Assembly Rooms at Surbiton. The patronage of Her Royal Highness, the Duchess of Teck, ensured its success and the *Sporting and Dramatic News* of 19 February, 1891 puts Dr and Mrs Langdon Down next to Lady Ellis as the main movers behind the event[15]. He was a generous man, both in spirit and in his support of worthy causes.

References

1 Normansfield account books, held by Mrs Patricia Langdon Down.
2 London Metropolitan Records Office. H29/NF/11/28/17[1].
3 London Metropolitan Records Office. LMRO; NF/B13/001.
4 The Bible. Old Testament, Revelations 5:13.
5 London Metropolitan Records Office. LMRO;A1/29/181.
6 London Metropolitan Records Office. LMRO;NF/B13/001.
7 JL Down. *The Education and Training of the Feeble in Mind.* London: HK Lewis, 1876.

8 Duncan PM, Millard WA. *Manual for the Classification, Training and Education of the Feeble Minded, Imbecile and Idiotic.* Longmans Green, 1866.
9 Andrew T. *Encyclopedia of Domestic Medicine and Surgery.* Glasgow: Blackie and Son, 1842.
10 Spensley FO. A brief account of Darenth and its system of industrial training. *J Ment Sc* 1913; **39**: 305–14.
11 *Christian Union.* 27 June, 1879.
12 Report. *BMJ* 1864; **2**: 416–18.
13 Report. *Lancet* 1869; **2**: 405–8.
14 Marvel W. *The Alabama and the Kearsarge.* Carolina: University of North Carolina Press, 1996.
15 *Sporting and Dramatic News.* 19 February, 1891.

Chapter 10

Development of Normansfield

Normansfield was a large house. Downstairs the dining room and drawing room were of elegant proportions; on the first floor there were two large rooms, one of which was subsequently converted into a billiard room; both of these probably functioned as mini-dormitories when the first patients came in. There were seven bedrooms and additional accommodation in the attic rooms. The boys were under supervision of a schoolmaster and two attendants, assisted occasionally by the coachman, who slept in a room with patients when required. There were clearly no demarcation disputes between the staff. The girls were under the care of a governess and six nurses. The ordinary pattern of care was for a group of residents to share a large room and to have a staff member to sleep with them, constituting a pattern of continuity, aimed at giving the residents a new sense of family. A single staff member, who today would be called a care worker was responsible for each sub-group of patients. Typically a sub-group consisted of three or more residents and their carer. Later some individual patients had their own designated carer and, at the top of the scale, some might have a whole villa assigned to them with separate staff. This would, of course, be an extra facility for which the family would be financially responsible.

Work started immediately on the building of the first part of the south wing. This contained 16 rooms and was completed by the summer of 1869, allowing for an increase in the number of patients and the transfer of some of the existing patients out of the main building[1]. Flower beds, lawns and walks were laid out in the grounds. Initially the patients were taken for exercise across the railway bridge into Bushy Park, or alternatively by waggonette, either to Bushy Park or Hampton Park. The foundation stone of the north block was laid on 15 July 1872, when the farm land and the River Field were also purchased and the completed north and south wings made it possible to increase the number of residents to 57. Adjacent villas were also purchased and these were used in the main for patients whose families were in a position to finance the extra staffing required. One villa was reserved as an infirmary in case of an epidemic. The importance of an infirmary for isolation of infected cases was something that Langdon Down had learned in his Earlswood days when he had dealt with the many major epidemics there. There were no effective treatments for many infections and the isolation of cases, particularly of scarlet fever, was a major requirement.

Langdon Down had, while in Earlswood, acquired some knowledge of farm management and Normansfield became a centre for pig production after farm buildings were built there in 1877. The Normansfield Large White became well-known and ultimately a herd of up to 150 pigs was reared. A herd of mainly Dexter cows was gradually added as well as this breed was hardy and healthy.

In 1877 work was begun on the new entertainment hall and central pavilion which took two years to complete. The architect was Rowland Plumbe, a friend of John Langdon Down's from 1853 whom he had met probably through church activities. As a medical student he had kept in touch with Rowland Plumbe and used to write to him to tell him about his examination results. Rowland Plumbe's son, Ebenezer, had been one of the first patients admitted by Langdon Down to the Earlswood Asylum. Their own affected child had alerted the Plumbes to the need for provision for services for the learning disabled. Mrs Plumbe had been one of the main movers in drawing the attention of the Reverend Andrew Reed to unmet needs in this field and the Plumbes had been associated with the development of Earlswood from its earliest days. Interestingly, when Langdon Down left Earlswood and many of the patients followed him, Ebenezer Plumbe remained where he had first been admitted.

The Earl of Devon formally opened the completed wings and theatre on 27 June, 1879[2] (see Chapter 12). It was a grand occasion, attended by, amongst others, the Presidents of the Royal College of Physicians, the Medico-Psychological Association, the Pharmaceutical Society, the Obstetrical Society and the Medical Society of London, the Master of the Worshipful Society of Apothecaries, and a broad cross section of the cream of scientific and social society of London.

It was in his opening address on this occasion that Langdon Down publicly acknowledged the strange moment of inspiration in which the sight of a feeble minded girl had activated in him the ambition to undertake the study of medicine and the amelioration of the lot of the learning disabled. He listed the countries from which residents were now being attracted – India, the West Indies, Siam, Persia, Australia, New Zealand, Germany, France and every part of the British Isles. The grounds had been extended to an area of 40 acres and the staff had grown to almost 100 in number[2].

Langdon Down's health had been affected by a serious illness in 1890 and he was confined to bed for three months. The pharmacy book shows him as having been on a quinine mixture, which was the standard treatment for high temperatures with infection. He did not sleep well, perhaps because of his cough or perhaps because he fretted at his inactivity. Bromide was added which he prescribed himself. Finally he went on to a digitalis mixture, suggesting that

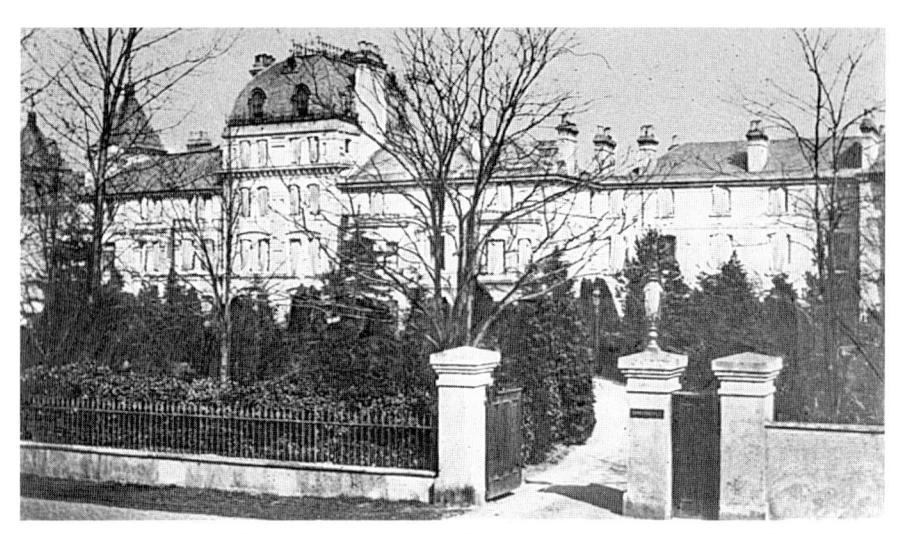

Normansfield, showing the extensive accommodation which was added to increase the number of admissions. At one stage there were 156 patients in residence, plus the Langdon Down family and staff.

there were cardiac complications. The evidence suggests he may have had severe influenza with subsequent cardiac failure. He returned to work but seemed prematurely aged. When he died in 1896 at the age of 68, the *Surrey Comet* described him as a venerable old man. He had exercised proper financial prudence and, in 1894, all his assets were put into a joint account with his wife Mary. In 1895, as an additional insurance, his two sons Reginald and Percival, both now medically qualified, were added to the Commissioners' Licence. Over the years Langdon Down had operated like a modern property developer, gradually assembling parcels of land and completed buildings so that, in the end, he was the owner of a large suburban estate. His access to the River Thames from his own property was to make it possible for him in later years to arrange for his guests to arrive by river boat. Both he and his sons had an enduring interest in the river and the Normansfield boathouse remains as a memorial to this special feature of the life of the Langdon Down family.

Of the 20 patients admitted in the first year, six were over the age of 20, pointing to a future problem of ensuring that discharges of older patients would make way for new admissions. Twelve of the patients were under the age of 15 and so might be described as being appropriately placed in a school programme. His programme of management, set out in *The Education and Training of the Feeble in Mind* first recommended a liberal diet. He drew attention to the importance of ensuring that the diet provided could be consumed by children who had poor development of chewing and swallowing. He realized how difficult it was to maintain a balanced diet when children had trouble with mastication. He placed great emphasis on the development of mouth and tongue control and on the provision of food which had been suitably prepared to meet their special needs.

The quality of the food in Normansfield could not be challenged. Mary Langdon Down made out the daily diet sheet herself and had a recipe book in which she wrote out recipes for the kitchen. When the Commissioners in Lunacy visited the hospital on 15 January, 1875 they described the diet as very good[3]. The Commissioners always visited without notice. On the day of the inspection there was a choice between beef or rabbit, apple pudding or cornflour and with the meal the residents could have 'wine, beer or water, according to the direction of Dr Down'. There was ample provision for providing a soft diet for those who needed it. Mary Down had a recipe for traditional panada, a bread and milk dish. Mincemeat was in such demand that a mechanical mincer had to be bought in 1889. These dishes were for the children who had difficulty in chewing and swallowing. All the residents had daily baths. Outdoor walks were emphasized and no opportunity was lost for daily outdoor activity. When the Normansfield grounds were fully developed the perimeter walk was over a mile long. Younger children played games in the Kindersaal under the theatre and a drill and exercise hall was built in 1879. Published brochures refer to tennis, croquet and cricket and there are photographs of Normansfield patients dressed for these and also for badminton, which was presumably played in the exercise hall.

As described in *The Education and Training for the Feeble in Mind*[4] Langdon Down found that in all imbeciles there is a lack of muscular coordination which he set out to improve by physical training. He paid special attention to the control of the lips and tongue and hoped to stop patients drooling as this was socially unacceptable. The Commissioners attested to the success of the training regime in their report of 8 October 1880, when they reported on the good deportment of the children at dinner, showing as they observed; 'what can be done by tact and judicious treatment to make imbecile children behave like rational beings[5]'.

The establishment of discipline in Normansfield was promoted through the development of a sense of responsive affection. The Rules for Officers, of which the 1888 draft survives, totally prohibit corporal punishment and restraint. Normansfield was to be run on family lines. To all the extended family, Mary Langdon Down was 'Little Mother'. The Langdon Downs lived under the same roof, walked in the same grounds, played the same games and shared the same activities as their residents. The attitude of the Langdon Down family was that if children came to live with them in their home it was because their parents had found it too difficult to manage them themselves and so they were to be incorporated into an extended family. The staff were expected to take their tone from the head of the institution which was one of affectionate regard for all the residents.

When patients were ill Langdon Down was in constant attendance. The Normansfield clinical records show the activities of a dedicated doctor. When Thomas M, a patient with spinal deformity and delusions, became terminally ill with bronchitis there was great anxiety about his condition. The notes show that Langdon Down was called and visited at 4 am and again at 6 am Unfortunately this patient died, but not from lack of medical care and attention[6]. When Mary Louise F developed burns from the ignition of her pinafore in 1876, Langdon Down visited her at midnight and found her comfortable. He visited her again at 1.30 am and adjusted her bandages because he thought they might need slackening. Unfortunately she too deteriorated and died[7]. The parents were, however, very appreciative of Langdon Down's efforts. As far as they were concerned 'everything was done that could be done for her and they will always have a grateful recollection of Dr Down's unremitting attention to her up to the last moment of her life... His behaviour was that of the good physician, who, if he could not cure, never ceased to care'[8].

A Family Home and Second Home

Normansfield was intended to be run like a family home accommodating an extended family. On 27 December, 1869 the Commissioners in Lunacy reported that all the residents, apart from those on leave and two who were ill, dined together on Christmas Day, with the attendants and nurses and some of the younger members of the Down family in attendance[9]. Very few residents went home and, indeed, for most of them Normansfield became their home from home. They enjoyed various games and amusements in the evening. This tradition of Christmas celebrations, at which every resident received a personal gift from Dr and Mrs Down, became firmly rooted. Every effort was made to try to ensure that the residents would enjoy the lifestyle which would have been their ordinary expectation within their family homes.

Residents went on excursions to Crystal Palace. At a later stage, staff reminisced about residents going to the pantomime in London in evening dress. On Sundays those who were judged fit attended Sunday Service in the theatre and for this the men and the boys were given flowers to wear in their buttonholes. There was church rehearsal on Thursday evening in the theatre. For church services a special backdrop had been painted. On one panel it had the text of the Lord's Prayer. In the centre, under the traditional scriptural Alpha and Omega letters was the text of Exodus, Chapter 20. This set out the directives of the Ten Commandments. On the third panel was the text of the Creed. The backdrop was used both to draw the attention of the residents to the rudiments of religion, but also to try to supplement the reading skills of those who were on the learning curve and advancing towards literacy. Repetition of the reading passages could promote their secular as well as religious education.

Residents of Normansfield were intended to live the lives of young ladies and gentlemen. They were recruited for cricket teams and involved in other sports, unlike in Earlswood, where only the staff were involved in the cricket matches. In the school room children were taught reading, writing and arithmetic. Written progress reports were sent to their parents. When the Commissioners visited on October 22, 1879, they found that those in the male school room were undergoing an examination by Mrs Down[10]. The inspectors found the boys to be of orderly demeanour and taking great interest in their school work. Some were writing copies very fairly and others were doing arithmetic or reading. In the view of the Commissioners the educational part of the children's training was not being neglected. On the same day the Commissioners found that in the Kindersaal the younger boys and a number of girls were at play and evidently enjoying themselves.

Normansfield as an institution attracted considerable public attention and was highly approved. In October 1877 the *Christian Union*, a religious paper, published an article describing Normansfield:

> In the pleasant country between Twickenham and Hampton Wick... an institution has been growing steadily for nine years which would probably rank among the most honourable, beneficial and fruitful outcomes of medical skill and philanthropy in England. That the Institution for the Feeble Minded at Normansfield should have been the work of one man, a consulting physician in the West End of London, rendered the success it has attained and the progress it is making all the more remarkable. With these convictions the writer purposes to record a recent visit to Normansfield...
>
> First as to the founder and master spirit of the Institution. It not infrequently happens to genial and earnest students of the healing art, in their familiarity with the manifold forms of human suffering, to conceive a sympathy or aptitude for some special form of disease or particular class of sufferers. It was so with Dr Langdon Down. When MB, with not a few medals, and studying hard for MD he happened to be on holiday in the west of England and was so impressed with the helplessness of an imbecile girl, so far in sympathy with her kind as to wait at table, that he thought if care and science could do anything for such miserables, he should try to do it. This thought never left him.
>
> Dr Down purchased Normansfield as a retreat outside but near the metropolis where he might hope to pursue his special

Development of Normansfield

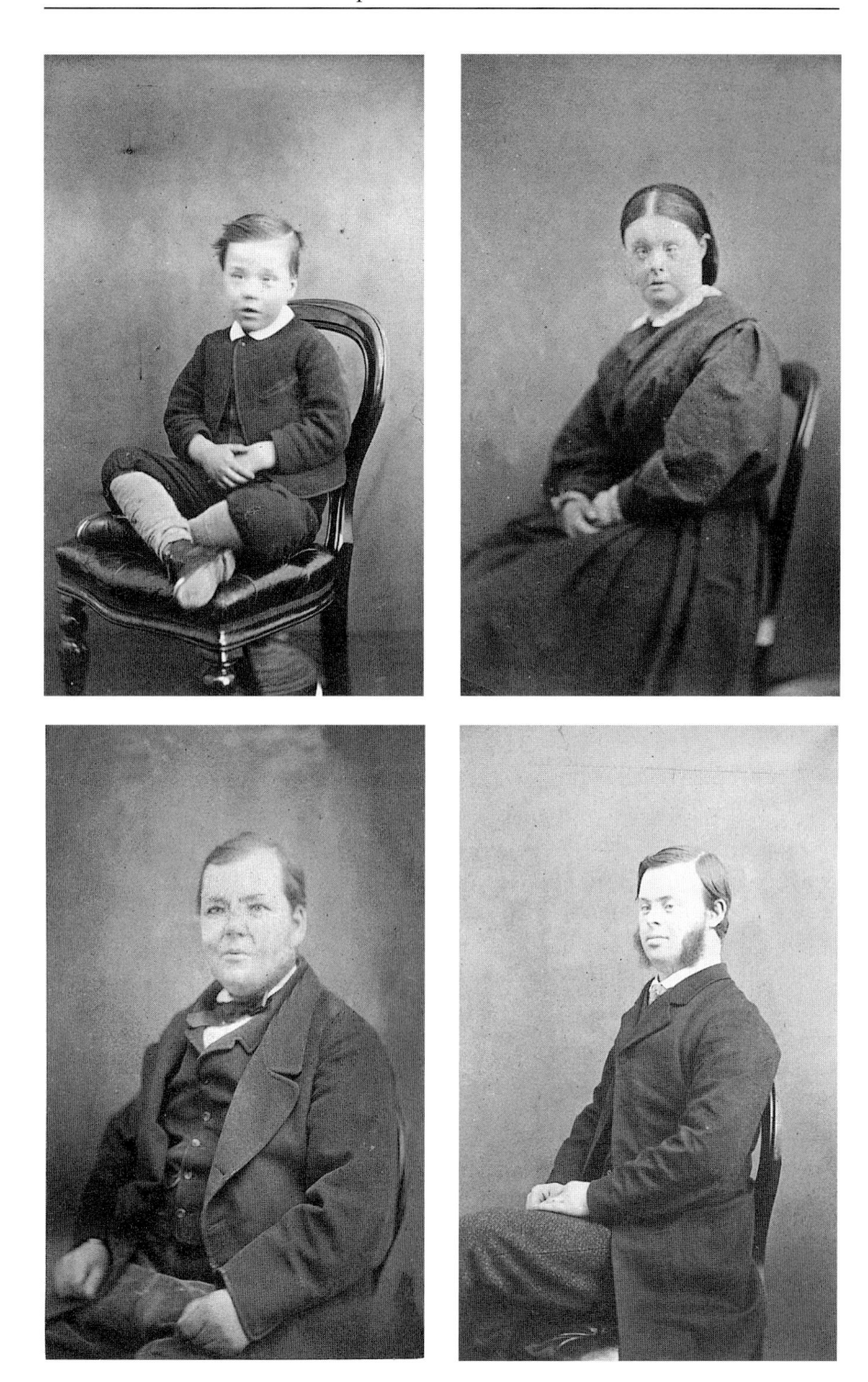

Four Down's syndrome patients. Part of the Earlswood series, photographed in 1865.

study... there are now 20 acres of ground laid off in lawns, garden and farm and walks and exercise grounds for the inmates, with a skill which leaves little to be desired. Seven or eight pupils in 1868 have increased to 108, in which number sexes are nearly equal... and who, male and female are all ages from three to twenty years or more. The boys and young men are domiciled in one wing of the buildings and the girls and children of either sex in another...

Everything done is of direct utility to the object of the institution. The sheep, the horses, the fowls, the gay plumaged birds, the agreeable variety of busy, orderly labour going on about the place, are all of the same piece as the cricket field, and the rare flowers and plants with which the lawns and the walks are adorned. They contribute to the health and happiness of the inmates, and form a part of the education by which the light of intellect is made to shine over their hitherto benumbed and beclouded senses.

The training process of Dr Down has its foundation in the corpore sano. Good health of the patients remains the first consideration; this end secured, the means of which in diet, regimen, cleanliness of person and clothing and the most skilful medical supervision are so minute and complete as seldom to fail, the mental training proceeds in an easy, natural and patient progress from what is simple to what is more compound, till in the repeated individual exercise, and the helping and stimulating companionship an example of others, the feeble faculties begin to operate, and will and action to respond to each other with more or less steady force...

Music has obviously the happiest effect on all this class of sufferers, of whatever age, or whatever degree of impotence not absolute. It is no little alleviation of their case that when they are alive to the inspiration and harmony of sweet sounds. One sees the almost ecstatic pleasure beaming in the countenances of the whole group, younger and older, when singing together with their teacher, and accompanist on the piano. But to account for the strength that music gives to the understanding, it seems that a group, thus singing together, bring into concentrative play the sense of mutual support and strength which forms a vital element of the general system at Normansfield. Each feels that he or she has contributed to a powerful result and in this experience finds a basis of new individual effort.

Of the mental education under Dr Down and the masters and governesses it may be said that, while adapting to the ages and various degrees of ability of the pupils, and to carry upward to considerable results, it is wholly free from the formality and rigour of the schools... The efficacy of the law of kindness has seldom been more strikingly illustrated that in this Institution for the feeble in mind. First perfect discipline is maintained without personal chastisement or material deprivation of any kind. No pupil is allowed to be shaken, or slapped, or deprived of necessary food, or subjected to any avengement. The duty laid on teachers and attendants is to gain the affection of their wards so fully that nothing will be to them a higher punishment than the disapprobation, or negative withdrawal of the love of their ministrants...

The Institution at Normansfield is necessarily reserved for the feeble and backward of the more wealthy classes, but the fact only suggests the question why the advantage of similar treatment should not be extended to the helpless offspring of the lower and more numerous ranks of society... Should not every county almost have an institution for imbeciles? Is there not a new question here for the state and for our legislators[11].

This glowing testimonial was repeated in the *Christian Union* on 27 June, 1879[12]. The editorial discussed the problems of the cause and cure of the feeble in mind and says that it is a matter which should concern all classes of society. It spoke of Langdon Down not drawing attention to the work which he himself had done, but endeavouring to demonstrate that the methods he used could produce results. The editorial also mentioned that he had given much time to a special committee of the Charity Organization Society which had been working towards the establishment of institutions for the poorer classes in which the Normansfield system could be applied with benefit.

The editorial spoke glowingly of Mary Langdon Down:

In this respect Dr Langdon Down has been ably assisted in his work by Mrs Langdon Down, who is pre-eminently a lady of Miss Florence Nightingale's type, being naturally of a sympathetic spirit, so devotedly winsome and loving in disposition as to be looked up to by every pupil with affection and simplicity. To our mind this is one of the great secrets of Dr Langdon Down's success in the treatment of his patients. Besides this, Normansfield is more like a home than a college or an institution. It has all the comforts and associations of a home, with the accompaniments of mental and medical training and treatment[12].

When John Langdon Down entertained guests at the International Medical Congress in 1881, the Congress of Hygiene in 1891 and the British Medical Association in 1895 the events were covered in both national broadsheets and medical journals[13–18]. Up to 500 guests attended these functions; they were entertained by military bands, orchestras and performers and dined on the gourmet selections of a French chef.

Normansfield had a good relationship with the community in general. It provided employment, used local resources and its accounts with local tradesmen were substantial. John Langdon Down was regarded as a generous man so it was with some surprise that he found himself challenged by the Local Board on a matter of hygiene. In 1889, the year in which he was elected as an Alderman of Middlesex, the Inspector of Nuisances reported that his attention had been drawn to sanitary defects; he found that dirty water from the laundry at Normansfield was pumped out onto land within 40 yards of a road. He subsequently also discovered that sewage from the ordinary cesspool from Normansfield was pumped out onto adjoining land usually between 6 am and 9 am. Notice was given to discontinue this practice but Dr Down objected[19].

Dr Gunther was the Medical Officer for the area. It must be conceded that he was now in a position in which there was a conflict of interest. His salary as Medical Officer was £36 per annum, but his income from Normansfield was much greater; two thirds of the admission certificates for Normansfield residents carried his signature. He was frequently called in consultation by John Langdon Down and also often deputised for him. He reported, after visiting the place, that the laundry water smelt of nothing but soap and that it posed no nuisance or risk of injury to health. The house drainage was pumped out within an eighth of a mile of the high road. There was no smell when he was there because they were not then pumping. The problem appeared to be that there was a regulation limiting the hours in which a cesspool could be emptied. The stipulated hours were from midnight until 6 am.

Dr Gunther and the Chairman visited Normansfield. They reported that the whole sewage of the premises was flushed into one great cesspool, with another beyond to receive the overflow, which was first chemically deodorized. The cesspool was open at the top but no odour from it could be perceived. The effluent was pumped out on to the land and, although it could not be said that there was absolutely no smell from it, clearly nothing could be perceived at any distance. It was perfectly out of the question that any nuisance could be caused by this to the neighbourhood. Dr Gunther reported that, even when the cesspool was stirred with a pole, there was no detectable smell from it.

The Clerk had already written to Dr Down about the matter and, with regret, he had felt compelled to say that the practice of emptying the cesspool during prohibited hours should be discontinued. The Council meeting was later attended by Langdon Down. He described the drainage system and undertook to ensure that any restriction imposed by the council would be adhered to. After a long and animated discussion on the general question and Dr Down's case in particular, it was resolved that the Clerk should now write to Dr Down and express the Board's gratification that no nuisance now existed. In 1895, the year before Langdon Down died, the laundry was linked to the new public drainage system; there were no further complaints from the local authority. The episode had created nothing more than a flutter.

Normansfield struck back and, in the Christmas pantomime, Reginald and Percival Langdon Down discoursed:

> They started the sewage works over the way;
> Impossible! – fact I assure you,
> And they smell most atrociously so people say,
> Impossible! – fact I assure you,
> But no, it can't be, for by rumour I hear,
> The sewage directors are ready to swear
> The odour is caused by the gasworks so near,
> Impossible! – fact I assure you[20].

This appears to have been a contest in which there were no winners or losers.

At the celebrations for Percival's coming of age, also in 1889, a family friend made a speech in which he described Normansfield as the twin child of the same parents, born at the same time, prospering evenly and growing in strength and beauty from day to day. He said that it had been a delight to those who had been on the spot to see a comfortable country house grow to its present enormous dimensions:

> Dr Down had not been able to make the blind see or the deaf hear, but he had been able to throw light upon slumbering intellects, and to bring forth from the darkness to which they seemed to be doomed, the lights of intelligence. That was no mean benefit to all humanity, because in doing that he had taught others to do the like, and from all parts of the world, most eminent members of his profession had come to learn how they could treat similar cases. No greater honour could be conferred upon any man, and it was to those who were his immediate neighbours, a great pleasure to be able to congratulate him upon the eminent success of his establishment[20].

References

1 Twickenham Records Office. Memorandum prepared by Dr Norman Langdon Down c.1955.
2 *Medical Times*. 28 June, 1879.
3 Commissioners in Lunacy. Report 15 January, 1875.
4 JL Down. *The Education and Training of the Feeble in Mind*. London: HK Lewis, 1876.
5 Commissioners in Lunacy. Report 8 October, 1887.

6 London Metropolitan Records Office. LMRO; H29/NF/B13/001. F7.
7 London Metropolitan Records Office. LMRO; H29/NF/B13/004. F90.
8 Normansfield 1876. Unpublished Correspondence.
9 Commissioners in Lunacy. Report 27.12.1869.
10 Commissioners in Lunacy. Report 22.10.1879.
11 *Christian Union*. 12 October, 1877.
12 *Christian Union*. 27 June, 1879.
13 *The Times*. 28 July, 1881.
14 *Lancet* 1881.
15 *The Medical Press and Circular*. 10 August, 1891.
16 *Kingston and Surbiton News*. 24 August, 1891.
17 *The Daily Telegraph*. 17 August, 1891.
18 *Daily Chronicle*. 17 August, 1891.
19 *Kingston Express*. 7 March, 1888.
20 Unpublished family papers.

Chapter 11

The Mistress of Normansfield

Mary Langdon Down had ventured into Earlswood as a young bride. Percival, her fourth child, was born the week after Normansfield opened. Her sons Everleigh and Reginald were aged two and six when she and her husband started the new venture. She clearly had a very busy family life.

When Normansfield opened in 1868 her husband, John Langdon Down, had three concerns. Apart from the development of Normansfield he had his work at the London Hospital and also his private practice. The burden of development in Normansfield initially fell mainly to his wife Mary. She showed a tremendous talent for organization. A unit of the size of Normansfield would today have a financial director, nursing administrator, catering officer, works manager, steward, personnel officer and public relations officer. Mary Langdon Down, now aged 39, was all of these. She bought furniture for the new bedrooms, shopping around for quotations for beds, lockers, commodes and wardrobes. She saw to the installation of internal telephones and fire hydrants and the instruction of staff in fire control and, on a daily basis, set out the menu and organized supplies.

Normansfield needed up to 50 gallons of milk a day and she arranged with a company in Devon to have it sent by rail to Hampton Wick Station where it was collected by the Normansfield milk cart. She bought in 60 tons of coal delivered by barge at Kingston and then taken by cart from the barge quay at Kingston to Normansfield. She negotiated with the Hampton Court Gas Company to get a reduction in the charges for gas. Her obituary in the *Surrey Comet* spoke of her powers of organization and grasp of detail:

> Hers was the master mind that directed and controlled every detail connected with the management and working of Normansfield from its very foundation up to the time of her death, which has led to its great success. She was kind, though firm in her dealings with those in her employ, and by all, was held in the highest regard while among those in her own social circle, she was justly esteemed for her many amiable qualities. She was known by everyone as 'Little Mother[1]'.

She set out guidelines to staff which had to be strictly followed:

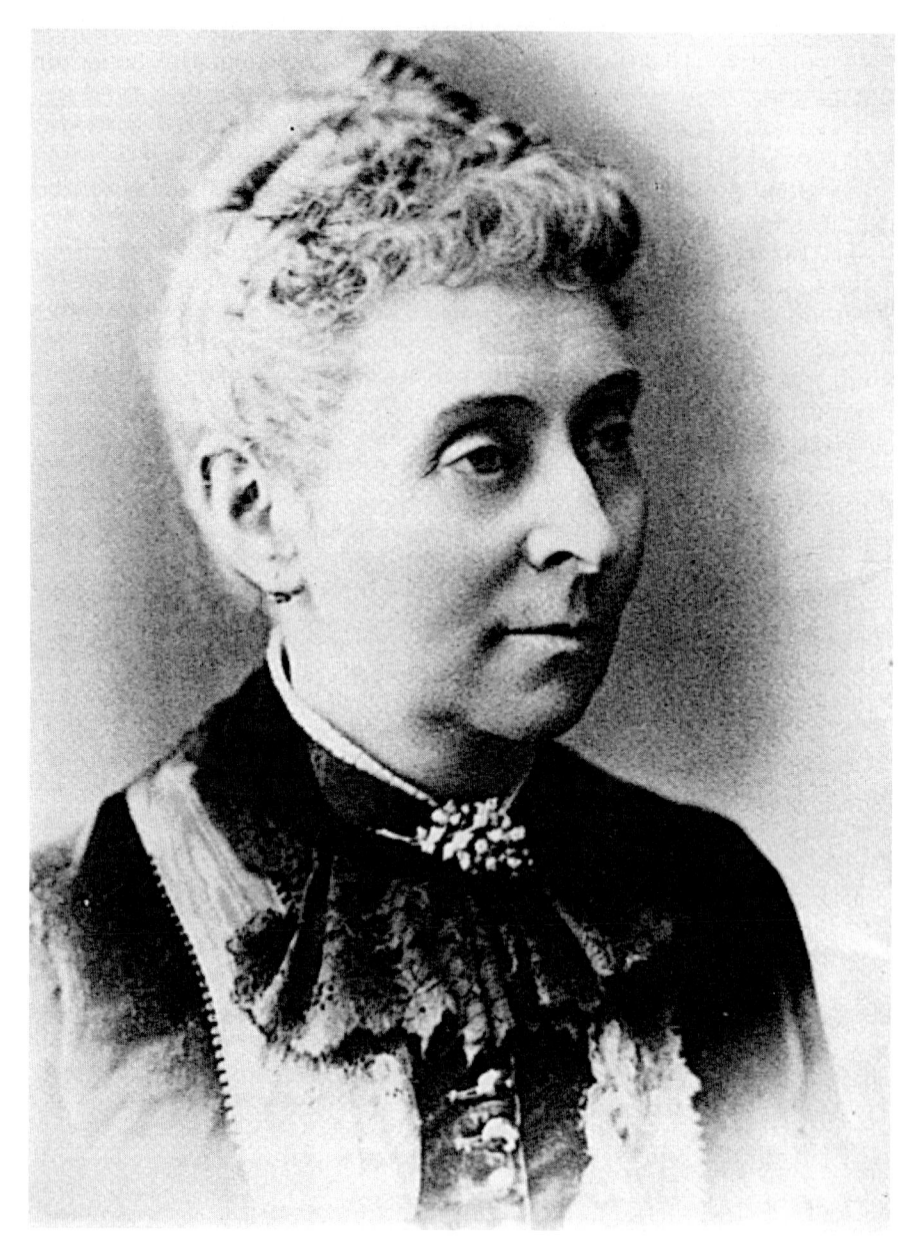

Mary Langdon Down at the age of 55, wearing the diamond brooch her husband bought her for their silver wedding. He paid £45 for it (£2,700 today).

The hour of rising is 6 a.m. It is not allowed to rise earlier without permission. All servants must be properly washed and dressed and be ready to commence duty at 6.30 a.m. The hour of leaving duty for nurses and attendants is 8 p.m. except for those whose turn it is to take evening duty. Servants must retire to their rooms by

10.15 p.m., be in bed and have the gas extinguished or lowered for the night by 10.30 p.m. Smoking is not allowed in the house or grounds. Tobacco and pipes must be kept where pupils cannot get at them and where they will not render the house offensive. Servants are strictly forbidden to inflict seclusion or restraint or punishment of any kind upon a pupil. A fine of 5 shillings will be given for breaking this rule. The second offence renders the servant liable to instant dismissal. If a pupil needs any correction it must be brought to the notice of the head of department or Mrs Langdon Down[2].

Patient Care

Mary Langdon Down's life was a busy one. In the administration of Normansfield she needed an administrative ability, tact, endurance and imagination. Parents trusted her and many of them wrote to her in informal terms, addressing her as 'My dear Mary'. They indeed saw her as being *in loco parentis*. She had many problems to cope with. Two boys from Ireland were on the waiting list for Harrow:

> A note from Mr Watson asking if Desmond is going to Harrow next term, and if so his present master's report as to his character, capacity and progress. I shall just write to say he will not be fit to go this year, that he has had whooping cough and that after that he was weak for some time and thrown back, is now improving and getting on... But we should like to know if anything more should be said or not. My husband adds that you will probably say it is too soon to specify anything. But in case we hear again from Mr Watson and you could tell us gently what to say, it would be a great help[3].

– here was a family facing up to the reality of special education; the parents sent the Langdon Downs a Christmas gift of two woodcock shot on their estate. During the festive season, letters came with presents for children. Mrs N wrote on 14 December, 1882:

My dear Mrs Langdon Down,

I have sent off a hamper for dear little Lucy, containing toys, books, dolls and a few eatables. I hope they will arrive safely and that she and the other little children will have a very happy day. I hope your children all keep well this very miserable weather. It must cause you very great anxiety having so many under your care at this time of year. I am looking forward to the arrival of Dr Langdon Down's letter. I am most anxious to know *his* opinion of my darling child.

Will you kindly give her this little note, with kind regards to the Dr and yourself.

Ever yours sincerely, Mary RN[3]

Another read: 'The 29th, Monday is Fred's twenty fourth birthday – can you manage some little treat for him – a drive or something of the kind. How are you all? I hope well – I can not get strong after the last operation I went through in the autumn. It takes too long'. Frederick had been in Normansfield fifteen years at that time[3].

The Normansfield residents varied in age from two years through to adults. There were more boys than girls, almost at a ratio of two to one; girls with a learning disability could probably be managed more easily at home. Boys tended to be admitted about two years earlier than girls, possibly because they had been more difficult to control at home or in temporary placements. The average age of admission was 11 for boys and 13 for girls.

Some admissions were due to the death of a parent or, in some cases, the death of both parents. Many parents could come to visit only once a year as they frequently lived abroad. English families who had settled on sheep farms in Australia or New Zealand found the management of children with learning disability to be beyond them. A Chief Justice in the British legal system in India had two sons in Normansfield and, for residents who were almost completely out of contact with their own families, it was up to Mary Langdon Down to provide a home from home for them. Residents sometimes came from other European countries and it must have been very challenging to deal with children who spoke only French or German when they arrived. The most challenging of all may have been a boy, described as being of Hebrew origin, whose parents were Moroccan and who spoke only Arabic.

Sometimes the admissions were related to unacceptable social conduct, which could prove to be particularly embarrassing when the eccentricity of behaviour conflicted specifically with the social role of the family. Some children had very special needs. Margaret B was blind, from congenital syphilis; Frances C had cataracts; George E had a hare lip and cleft palate and many had cerebral palsy of one form or another. George B had been born in Siam of English parents; he understood what was said to him in Siamese but not in English and he had acquired several vulgar Siamese habits which are not specified in the records. He made little progress with his education but developed an interest in gardening and appears to have been happy in his work.

Francis P, aged 9, was reputed to practise masturbation 20 times a day. He had played indecently with his younger brother and had thoroughly corrupted his sister. He had also been guilty of the grossest sensuality with the female servants. Dr Down prescribed ablution of his genitals with iced water and he was discharged one year later with a note to say that he was 'recovered'. Langton EB was the son of a vicar who had taken to undressing himself in the churchyard when the congregation were leaving church. He was described on admission as having no bruises on his body, possibly to be taken as portraying his father as a tolerant man. He too was discharged improved and with the hope that he might be tried at an ordinary school.

Some of the older patients must have caused her concern. Dickson JC, aged 21, had been troublesome at the school and had not been able to learn like other boys. He was tried in his father's counting house but nothing could be done with him. He had been sent from tutor to tutor, making no progress. He was restless and morose and went through a phase of hyper-excitability, which did not improve on bromide, supplemented by chloral at night. One attendant could not control him and, in the end, four men had to be called and contrary to general policy, he had to be restrained by a camisole, with his legs secured by towels. He was discharged the following day, being one of the few patients in whom the moral treatment advocated by Langdon Down had failed. With her husband Mary was frequently called upon to be with patients in their last stages, as when Katherine MS died on 20 June, 1882 at 2.20 in the morning. Katherine's mother had been summoned and was consoled as best they could by the Langdon Downs. When Mary's husband was called at night she frequently went with him. At least their patients were all close by.

Social Events

Mary was also the hostess at a number of major events which required great organization. For the opening of the new wings and the Theatre in 1879, 200 guests were entertained. The band of the Grenadier Guards was engaged to provide background music. Outside caterers were brought in and, on this occasion, luncheon was served in the recreation hall. Normansfield was the setting for a number of such large social functions.

When the International Medical Congress was held in London in August 1881, three large receptions were held in honour of the visitors. One was hosted by Mr Spencer Wells, President of the Royal College of Surgeons, one by Baroness Coutts, of the banking family and the third and possibly the largest by Dr and Mrs Langdon Down. As a precaution, Mary Langdon Down had arranged with an outside caterer to provide for up to 800 guests. Once more, the band of the Grenadier Guards had been engaged and, on this occasion, the Royal Handbell Ringers as well. The attendance included the world famous Abraham Jacobi and Samuel Gee, as well as other famous figures. Langdon Down was not,

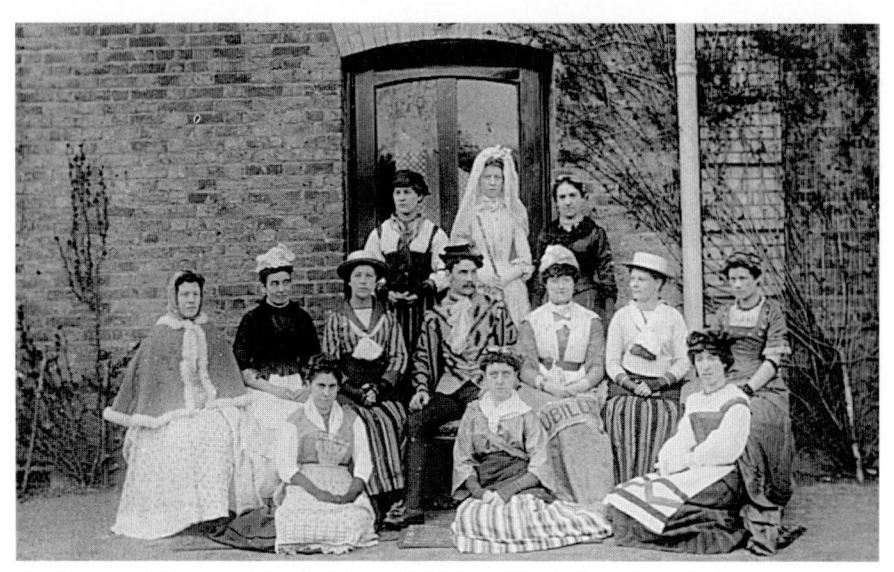

The Normansfield pageant for the Diamond Jubilee of Queen Victoria in 1897.

however, to the fore in the scientific programme and did not make any medical contribution to the meeting.

The biggest celebration of all was held in 1889 when Percival, the Langdon Down's youngest son, reached the age of 21. The occasion coincided with the postponed celebration of the Jubilee of Queen Victoria (see Chapter 15). These social events represented great challenges. They received widespread coverage in the press and many tributes were paid to Mrs Down[4].

Financial Management

The serious business of making Normansfield a financial success depended on striking the right balance between income and expenditure. The scale of charges to residents varied according to their specific needs. In 1880 the total fee income was £12,241. This year has been chosen as a typical year for financial analysis at a time when Normansfield had proved itself in the market place[5]. There were 77 residents, whose families paid an annual charge ranging from 60 guineas at the bottom end of the scale to 300 guineas at the top end; the annual average charge was 129 guineas, £7740 at current money values. This could not be regarded as excessive for the standard of care provided, and the range of charges corresponded to the Earlswood Asylum scale for upper-class residents. In 1883, a comparable year for which the information is available, there were 19 officers on the staff, with 52 female servants and 25 male servants, of whom 10 were gardeners and labourers. The sheer size of the property clearly required that there should be a substantial workforce. Of all the officers, the chaplain was the highest paid at £100 per annum, followed by the headmaster at £80. At the lower end of the scale female servants were paid £15 per annum and male servants £24 per annum.

With the overall income of Normansfield running at over £12,000 per annum, salaries at £2,200, food and other bills at £900 per annum, gas £200 and servicing of debt £1700, it was possible to assign approximately £5000 to the sinking fund. On this basis year by year, the overall debt was gradually cleared. John and Mary Langdon Down drew no salaries from Normansfield nor did any of the Langdon Down family in later years. In Ticehurst, the private psychiatric institution, the Newington doctors drew salaries of £1800, the equivalent of £108,000 today. The Langdon Down family, by contrast, applied their surplus income to the reduction of the Normansfield debt.

As far as staff were concerned, leave was strictly controlled. Staff were entitled to 28 days' leave in all, but half days taken during the week were deducted from the annual leave allowance. There was no afternoon leave allowance. Attendants rose with their patients, prayed, worked and slept with their allocated charges. Their own entertainment and that of the residents was all arranged on site; in addition to all her other duties Mary also played a great part in organizing this at Normansfield (see Chapter 12).

Education and Affection

Mary Langdon Down was an extraordinary woman. There was almost no higher education for women but Mary had studied hard. She had set herself to learn what she could about household and institutional management and read an enormous amount, ranging from economic science to physiology, from beekeeping and poultry-rearing to household management. She took her religious studies seriously and her own copy of Butler's *Analogy of Religion* is thumbed and underlined. Hopley's *Plain and Simple Lectures* on the education of man were also in her library of books; he was to the fore in naming wrongs which cried for redress and chastised governments for the neglect of public hygiene, poor conditions in factories and other evils[6]. She was probably the author of the long fund-raising poem entitled *The Idiot*, a eulogy of Earlswood published anonymously in 1865[7].

These were not the interests of an isolated bluestocking, isolated from the hardships of the real world. In character she was warm, interested, and friendly. Whenever there was an admission to Normansfield she sat and made her own notes on likes and dislikes, established bedtime rituals, fears and phobias, comforts and concerns. Her husband was never 'Dear Langdon', or 'Dear John'. He was 'Dearest' or 'My Dearest'. A woman who, in her portrait, could be described as handsome rather than beautiful, her warm personality sustained both her husband and their joint enterprise. She put little surprise notes in his bag when he set out for London. A few have survived, including one written on 11 April 1890:

> Dearest,
>
> You had better answer this. I am delighted that you are having such a beautiful day for going to the hospital. You will never know how much you mean to me.
>
> All my love, Mary[8].

She kept the back issues of *The Family Economist*, filed its recipes and studied its homespun philosophy and educational features. A passage which she marked described the good wife: 'The good wife would not cross her husband in the springtime of his anger but would stay until it ebbed'[9]. She could ignore this instruction as her husband was a patient and tolerant man. 'If a husband were away a good wife would double the toil of her diligence'[10] – this indeed she did. His hospital and practice kept her husband away from Normansfield for most of the day but, because of Mary, he could look forward to peace and order on his return.

References

1. *Surrey Comet.* 7 October, 1901.
2. Rules to be observed by the Officers of the Establishment, Normansfield 1888.
3. London Metropolitan Records Office. LMROH29/NF/A1/29/417.
4. *Kingston and Surbiton News.* 6 July, 1889.
5. Normansfield Account Books. Courtesy of Mrs Patricia Langdon Down.
6. Hopley T. *Plain and Simple Lectures on the Education of Man.* Lecture **3**(suppl): 41–60. London: Houlston, Wright, 1858.
7. Anon. *The Idiot.* London: Allingham, 1865.
8. London Metropolitan Records Office. LMRO; NF/A/01/053.
9. *The Family Economist.* London: Groonbridge & Sons, 1848: 16.
10. *The Family Economist.* London: Groonbridge & Sons, 1848: 43.

Chapter 12

Sundays, Weekdays and Entertainment

The Normansfield Theatre

The need for a recreation centre led to plans for a building of a two-storey hall, the lower floor of which was to be a children's kindersaal or recreation room and the upper floor the Normansfield theatre. Before leaving Earlswood the Langdon Downs' last formal appearance had been at an entertainment for patients at which Dr Langdon Down's 'Prologue to a Concert' had been delivered by Mary Langdon Down herself. Now, in their own centre, they were to take in hand the organization of recreation and entertainment on a regular basis. They were experienced and talented and the Normansfield entertainments not only engaged the attention of staff and patients but also the general public, who were invited to special performances, especially at the New Year. These attracted very flattering reviews in the local papers[1].

The Normansfield theatre, opened in 1879, had been designed to fulfil two functions. It was to be an entertainment centre and a church. *Crockford's*[2] has no entry relating to a chaplain until 1884 and, in the intervening years, the chaplaincy arrangements were made informally with the parish church. The chaplain was probably the vicar of Hampton Wick. The first full-time chaplain, appointed in 1883, was Nonconformist. In 1884, the year after Everleigh's death, the first Church of England chaplain was appointed. When it was necessary to close Hampton Wick parish church for repairs in 1879 the congregation attended Sunday service in the theatre in Normansfield.

The Sunday service was an important event in the week's activities. Before Normansfield had its own chaplain, residents who were fit to do so attended morning service in Hampton Wick. The records for 1871 show that 17 out of the 37 residents were listed on a Sunday service register. Retaining the attention of a rather restless congregation must have taxed the communication skills of the chaplains and, in 1882, the official Visitors recommended that the sermons should not exceed 10 minutes in length.

Rehearsal for Sunday service was held on Thursday evenings. Residents practised hymns, the Lord's Prayer, the Creed and the Ten commandments. A backdrop on the theatre stage spelt out the words. Residents could practise their spelling and reading at the rehearsals. To be allowed to attend a Sunday service was a privilege; women and girls wore their best dresses and the men were all supplied with

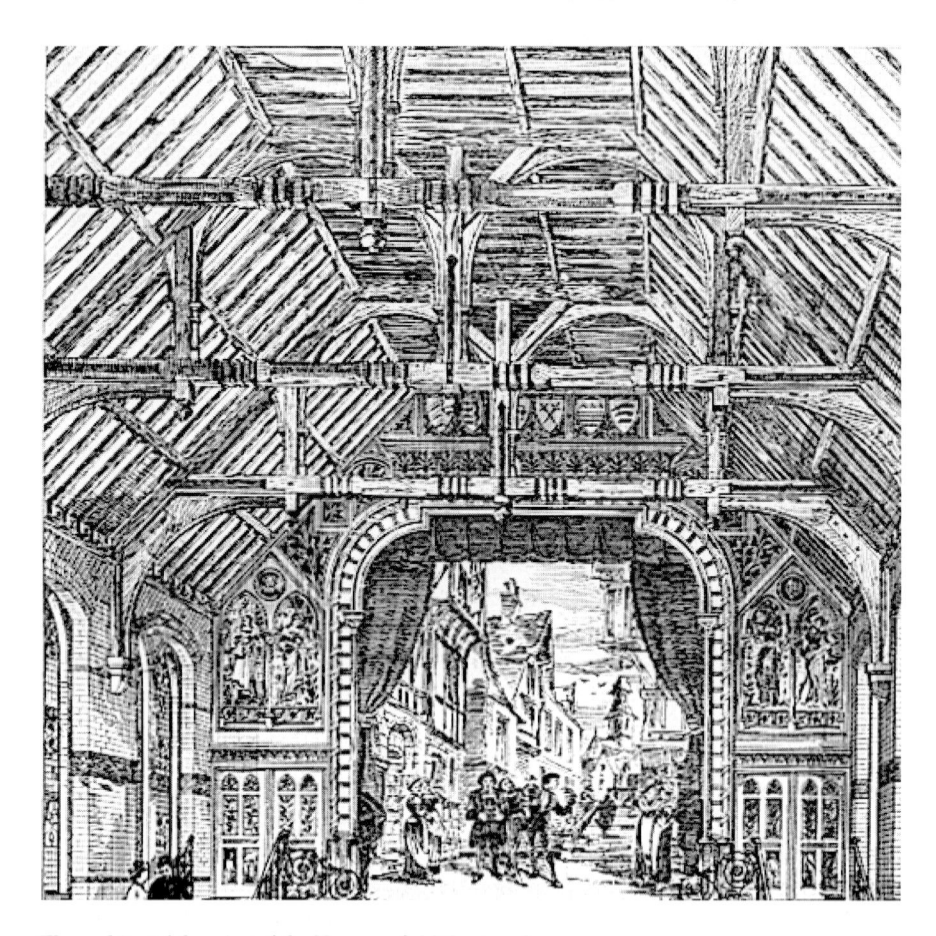

The architects' drawing of the Normansfield theatre plan.

a flower for their buttonholes. Langdon Down hung a symbolic painting on the wall of the theatre. Attributed to Tintoretto, it showed the lame man healed by Christ at the pool of Bethesda. The sick had gathered to await the rippling of the water by the angel of the Lord and the lame man had missed his chance to climb into the pool. The miracle of the healing of disability reflected Langdon Down's belief and he wished to make a point.

A Family Concern

Thursday evening was concert time and every resident who could sing or recite was encouraged to perform. In addition concerts were given by the Normansfield orchestra and band. There was an organ and a piano in the theatre. At Christmas time there was always a special performance of a pantomime, written by Langdon Down and his wife. Mary was very involved in the provision of entertainment for the patients, an interest that had begun at Earlswood. Once the theatre had been built she became the stage manager. She and her husband cooperated in staging entertainments and the family members were conscripted, or perhaps volunteered, to take part in plays and cabarets. Reginald, Percival and the ill-fated Everleigh all featured in the Christmas entertainment of 1874. Mary and John had together written a prologue which was delivered by Langdon Down himself:

> It is not a nameless pleasure we pursue:
> Much higher purposes we have in due;
> To wake the senses stricken in their birth;
> To rouse dull apathy in harmless mirth,
> To fix the attention by word or by sound,
> To bring back reason at a single bound:
> To pacify the irritable child, and watch the
> sufferer of its pain beguiled,
> To bring the light into the vacant eye,
> and cheer the heart of those more prone to cry:
> Distract the thoughts of those who pine for home,
> and touch some chord in minds that seem o'erthrown.
> For soothing care that all misfortunes bring
> We feel with Hamlet that 'the play's the thing'[3].

In 1889 Reginald and Percival, now close to completing their medical courses, performed a topical duet together which they had specially written for the occasion. The *Kingston Express* described the event, mentioning Mary's role and also drawing attention to the fact that 'Langdon Down, as he is well known, makes the provision of healthy recreation for his patients an important factor in his very successful method of treatment and the possession of histrionic ability, to be devoted to this end, is by no means the least important of the qualifications required in those who form part of the staff'[4]. When the Genesta Dramatic Club was organized, Mary Langdon Down remained active on the committee up to the time of her husband's death. The history of the Normansfield Theatre and the dramatic activities is given in full in the appendix contributed by John Earl (Appendix 2).

Reginald and Percival both inherited their parent's interest in the theatre and continued to show interest in the stage in later life. Percival had appeared in the Cambridge Footlights Dramatic Club productions while he was a student. Reginald and Percival's 1889 duet ended with a telling couplet:

> Squire – our inmates are happy in spite of their ills;
> Impossible! – fact, I assure you.
> Hugely we find music and dancing
> much better than pills.

Impossible! – fact, I assure you.
Squire, we need not at Normansfield bolts, bars and locks,
we've only to put a new play on the stocks,
our show is worth more than a guinea a box.
Impossible! – fact, I assure you[4].

This indeed was their parents' attitude and they worked hard to provide regular entertainment for the residents and staff.

Attendants recruited through employment agencies had to have some entertainment skills and it was Mary's job to ensure that all the Normansfield staff were suitably qualified in this respect. Hill and Courtneys bureau regretted in December 1897 that they had not been able to send a musician attendant to Normansfield and, in the

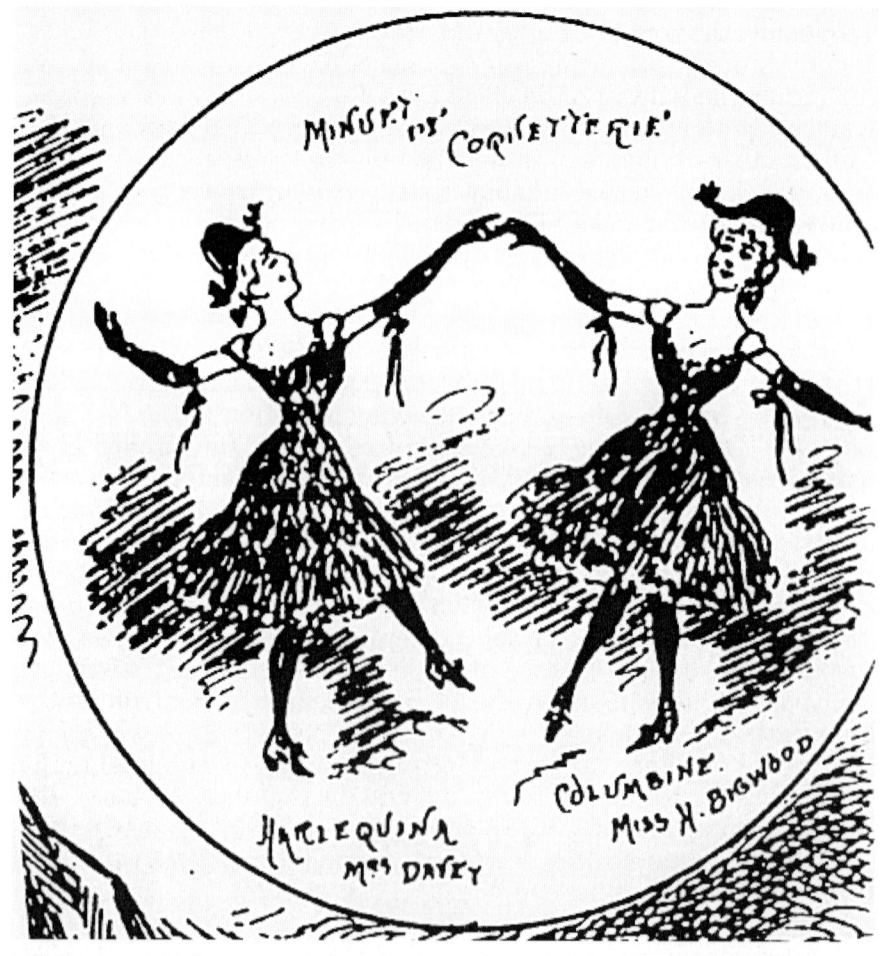

The Normansfield theatre was host to the Genesta Amateur Dramatic Club, with which the Langdon Down family were associated. The Illustrated Sporting and Dramatic News of 16 January 1893 shows Miss M Bigwood in the role of Columbine. She later married Dr Percival Langdon Down.

month of February, apologized for the fact that they did not have a violin player on their books[5]. They did, however, have a clean, smart young man who was well up in stage management, setting up entertainments, minstrel shows etc and who might be a suitable recruit. All staff should be able to either play an instrument or sing; one assistant master recruited on the basis that he could also play the organ lost his job when it turned out that his organ playing was below standard. Relationships with the staff, however, were always good and many completed 20 years' service, always recognized by a public presentation. Two in fact served Normansfield for 50 years.

In addition to the theatre there was a tennis court in Normansfield, which was used by the family and the more advanced patients. Badminton was played in the drill hall and, outside, the girls played croquet and the boys cricket. There were organized sports days in the summer with competing teams. On summer days they were taken into Bushy Park; here they saw the deer and collected antlers in the woods. Residents who had their own horses could have them groomed and stabled; others cycled or were taught to row. Craftsmen welcomed residents in the three workshops; some helped in the garden and some with the farm animals.

Christmas Festivities

The highlight of Normansfield's social calendar was the Christmas pantomime. Christmas was celebrated with great enthusiasm; apart

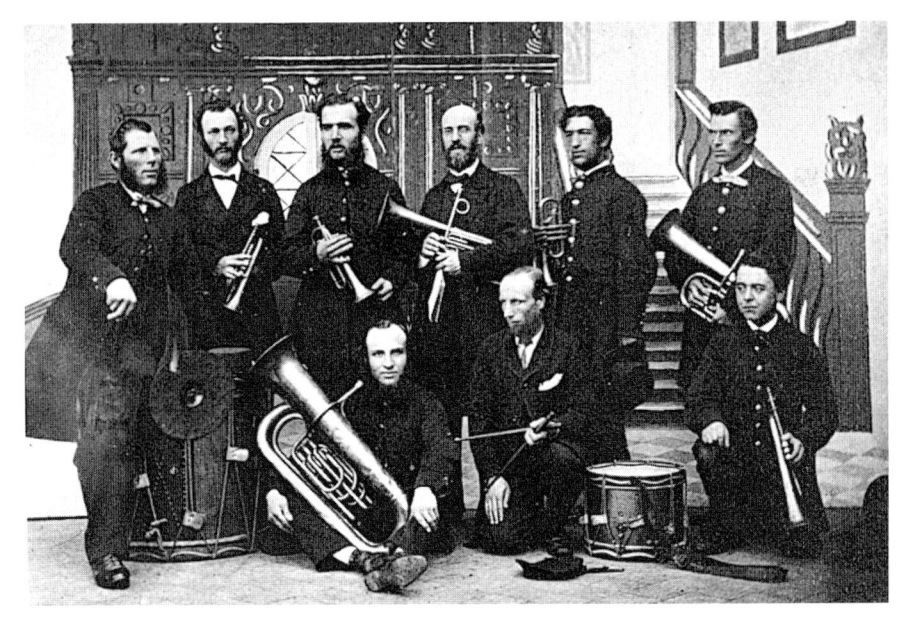

Every new member of staff was required to have musical or entertaining skills. Normansfield had an orchestra and a band made up of staff members. The photograph is from 1895.

from presents from their own families all the residents were given an individual present by the Langdon Downs. A Christmas tree was brightly decorated and on Christmas Day residents who had not gone home were joined for dinner by the Langdon Down family. The pantomime was repeated on two successive evenings for the residents of Hampton Wick and the theatre was packed to the doors on these occasions. The orchestra went from strength to strength and, ultimately, there were 16 members. The concert in 1887 opened with a musical selection at which Langdon Down mounted the stage and addressed the audience: 'I have been requested to speak a prologue which has been composed by a member of our staff, who is also a member of the band. It is as follows:

> Good friends – another year has gone; time flies apace,
> One more we welcome here each smiling face,
> In hope, by every art within our power
> To banish care and pass a cheerful hour
> And if our poor endeavours to amuse
> Should meet your favour, please do not refuse
> Your kind applause
> Thus much we dare to ask:
> Each effort then will be a cheerful task
> But – so the poets say (nor woman either)
> Hence our little play
> May have its faults and fail to please your taste
> If so, we ask you not chide in haste
> But let the will be taken for the deed
> and kindly prove yourselves true friends in need
> May this new year to you fresh blessings yield
> This is the wish of all at Normansfield[6].

There followed three sketches in which parts were taken by teachers, attendants and other staff. Between the sketches there were further vocal items and, as the local press reported, the programme had been, 'as usual of capital quality, with no barren intervals, well-staged, well-dressed and overall deserving of all praise'[6]. The Langdon Downs fostered an amateur dramatic society, the Genesta Club, which rapidly developed a membership of over 200. The Genesta players also contributed to the Normansfield entertainments and were ultimately able not only to stage plays, but also light opera.

Social Entertaining

Apart from the development of Normansfield, Dr and Mrs Down quickly became involved in the local social scene. They entertained and were entertained by their titled neighbours. When John

Langdon Down moved from his rented consulting rooms in Welbeck Street to his newly leased premises in Harley Street, the family also became involved in many social events in London. They attended social occasions in Harley Street, Fitzroy Street and at Broom Hall in Teddington. Their closest Teddington friend was Sir Thomas Nelson, solicitor to the City of London.

The Langdon Downs were genial hosts. He was at his best when he sat at the head of a generous table and Mary's charm made many friends for both of them. In London Langdon Down became a member of the prestigious Athenaeum Club and a member of the Broderers' Company, a Livery Company of the City of London. Many years later, in 1889, he was elected auditor of the Company, a high honour.

References

1 *Kingston and Surbiton News.* 24 January, 1885
2 *Crockford's Clerical Directory.* London, 1884.
3 Unpublished family papers, courtesy of Mrs Patricia Langdon Down.
4 *Kingston and Surbiton News.* 12 January, 1890.
5 London Metropolitan Records Office. LMRO29/NF/AL/28.
6 *Kingston and Surbiton News.* 22 January, 1887.

Chapter 13

A Death in the Family

Langdon Down and Mary travelled frequently to the Continent. They had medical friends whom they often visited, especially in Paris. On Saturday 4 August 1883 they set out at 6 am to catch the boat-train. Percival, their younger son who was always very close to his parents, travelled with them to London. Everleigh, now aged 21, and Reginald, aged 17, were at home, Reginald having returned on vacation from Harrow School. Everleigh had not been to public school and, in fact, it has not been possible to trace where he was educated and it remains something of a mystery. He did not go to Harrow like his younger brothers. A book of the collected works of Shakespeare was given to him by a Herbert Taylor Ottley, with a Charterhouse address. The Charterhouse records, however, do not identify Langdon Down as a pupil there. Everleigh did not proceed to higher education for a profession and when he died nothing was said of him except that he had planned a career in the army. He was a lieutenant in the Surrey Militia, perhaps with the idea that part-time military training might later lead on to a formal military career. Although the eldest of the family he was not his parents' favourite. His brothers' coming of age parties were lavish. His seems to have passed unnoticed.

In 1881 he was lodging with a Mrs Lankester in Hampstead, the widow of Dr Edwin Lankester, who had been London City Coroner from 1862; she was an author of books on British wild flowers. There would seem to be no good reason for Everleigh to be in lodgings in London, as he could easily have been accommodated in 81 Harley Street. The fact that he had not attended a second level school raises the question of his possibly having been dyslexic and he may have been a resident pupil of Mrs Lankester's. Overall there was an impression in the family that Everleigh did not share the academic interests of his younger brothers, both of whom were doing very well at school. In his death notice Everleigh was listed as living at Harley Street; he may have moved out from the Lankester home in the previous year.

He had become an officer in the 23rd Surrey Militia and may have needed help in meeting the army recruitment requirements. The Militia was a local part-time defence force and he may have looked on his part-time commission as a first step on the road towards a career as a regular army officer. Another possiblity is that he had an association with one of the military bands. The band of the 3rd

Militia was sometimes engaged to provide background music at social functions at Normansfield. Perhaps his regiment, the 23rd, also had a band in which he could exercise the family musical talent.

The local newspapers reported the sad course of subsequent events[1]. After breakfast Everleigh and Reginald went into the carpenter's shop. Reginald was already a skilled craftsman and, when older, built a boat with his brother Percival which they sailed together. Everleigh, however, was more interested in fishing. The brothers got on quite well together but this time they had a disagreement. Reginald set about turning a piece of brass on a lathe but Everleigh wanted to get out on the river. He exploded, snatched Reginald's brass, threw it on the floor and hit it again and again with a hammer. Reginald was understandably angry and upset and James Bradley, the senior Normansfield carpenter, tried to intervene. Reginald kicked Everleigh in the shin. What happened next is unclear. A large one and a half inch chisel lay on the bench beside Reginald. Bradley had laid the chisel to his right and Everleigh stood to his left. Suddenly Everleigh fell to the floor, bleeding so severely from his groin that the blood gushed through his clothes on to the shavings on the floor. Bradley had not seen the chisel pass in front of him. This was a heavy paring chisel; if Reginald threw it and it bounced off the bench and struck Everleigh a glancing blow Bradley should have heard it, and he did not.

The bleeding was torrential. Dr Gunther was sent for urgently and arrived in half an hour. Everleigh was, by now, bled white and Dr Gunther stopped further bleeding by pressing firmly on the groin.

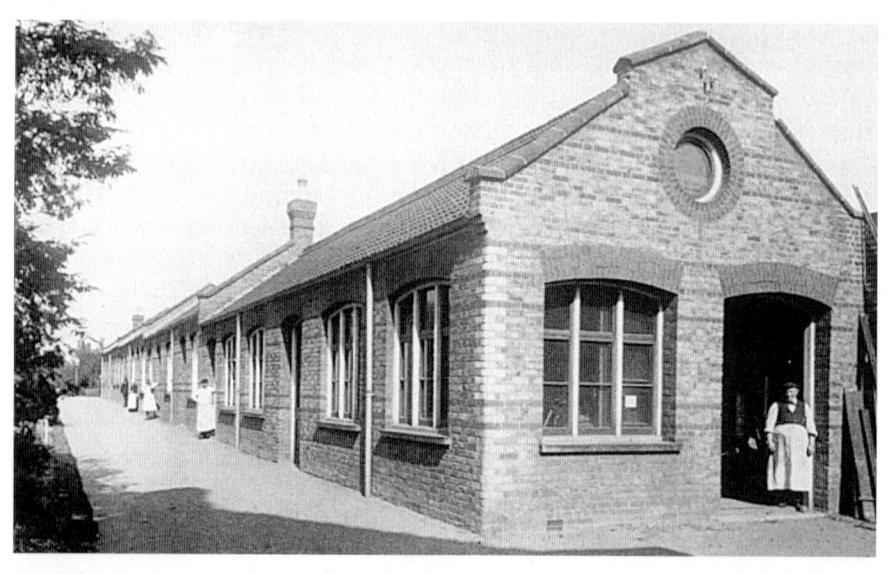

The Normansfield workshops. The nearest is the carpentry shop where Everleigh died; the furthest away is the pharmacy. A photographic dark-room was partitioned off the back of the pharmacy.

He then applied a tourniquet and sent for Mr Hutchinson, the senior surgeon at the London Hospital. Everleigh was still conscious and was upset when he was told that it could be a full year before he rode a horse again. He might indeed have to think again about something other than the army. It was 3 pm when Mr Hutchinson arrived. He explored the gaping wound and discovered that, beneath the inch-long gash, the tissues were widely incised. The sartorius muscle was completely severed and the femoral artery and vein were cut across as well as the adductor muscle. He tied all the cut blood vessels, closed the wound and left for London.

Dr Gunther called in two local medical men, Mr Farr White and Dr Farmer. Everleigh came around from the choloroform but was very weak and no pulse could be felt at the wrist. He was too ill to be left and the three doctors arranged a rota between them to cover constant attendance over the next 24 hours. Dr Farmer was due to stay with him first but Dr Gunther and Mr Farr White remained close by in the dining room. At 5.10 pm Dr Farmer sent a message to them saying that Everleigh was dying. They rushed back and found him unconscious and collapsed. A brandy enema failed to revive him and he died quickly.

Dr Gunther contacted the coroner, Dr Diplock. He called an inquest for Monday 6th August, 1883[1]. The distraught parents were called back from Paris by telegram and arrived the next day. The inquest was held in the Normansfield dining room. John Langdon Down sat to one side with his friend Sir Thomas Nelson, the solicitor for the City of London, and was very distressed.

The jury was enlisted and, having heard the medical evidence, two carpenters were put on the stand – James Bradley, who had been at the same bench as the brothers, and Charles Roach, who had been kneeling behind the bench. The Langdon Down family was represented by a London solicitor, Mr Humphries. James Bradley stated that when Everleigh fell down he called out: 'I am done for'. Reginald had said that he was very sorry that he had done it. Everleigh had replied: 'It is not your fault – I am to blame'. Charles Roach remembered that he had told James Everett, the chief attendant, that he had heard Reginald say: 'I did not intend to hit him'. James Bradley could not say whether the chisel had been thrust in or thrown, but it was clear that Everleigh had not asked for the chisel to be passed to him.

Dr Diplock summed up. There was no doubt, he said, that Everleigh had received a wound in the thigh which had divided his blood vessels and that his death was due to the resulting haemorrhage. Dr Gunther had raised the possibility that his death might have been due to a blood clot in the heart but, if this were so, the clot would have been a result of the haemorrhage. If the chisel had been thrown by Reginald with the intention of causing injury it would have been either manslaugher or murder according to whether or not it was done deliberately or in the heat of the moment. He put two questions to the jury: first, Did the chisel bound off the bench accidentally? and second, Was it thrown at the deceased purposely, and if so, by whom?

The jury deliberated for 10 minutes and returned a verdict of accidental death. This was a considerate and humane decision. The

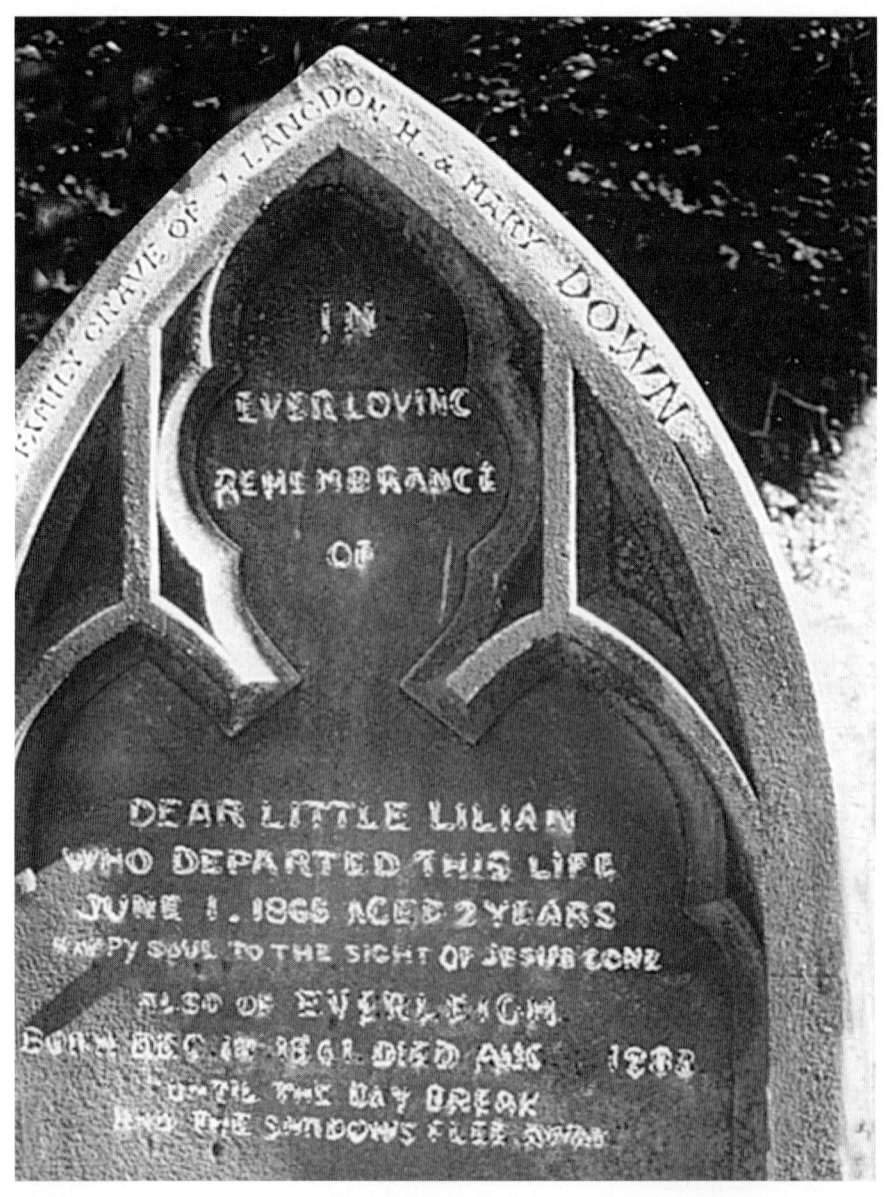

The tombstone in the Nonconformist plot in Redhill cemetery, where Lilian was buried in 1865 and Everleigh in 1883. The inscription on the headstone describes the plot as the family grave of Langdon H and Mary Down, but only Lilian and Everleigh were buried there.

Langdon Down family were well-loved and respected in the district and no jury would wish to add to their distress nor to burden a 17-year-old with long-lasting guilt for the fatal consequences of a hasty action. Everleigh's death notice read: 'Down, Aug. 4th at Normansfield, Hampton Wick, from an accident, Everleigh, eldest son of J. Langdon Down, MD, FRCP, of 81 Harley Street, aged 22 years'[2]. Dr Gunther had not informed the police and, in the circumstances, no statement had been taken from either Everleigh or Reginald. Dr Gunther was a friend and colleague; he justified his decision not to inform the police on the basis of not expecting the injury to prove fatal.

In retrospect it is clear that Everleigh provoked his brother when he kicked him. It was also unfortunate that Reginald had called his older brother a fool, perhaps in doing so releasing Everleigh's pent-up feeling of jealously at Reginald's good academic progress, which he himself could not match. Everleigh was, to a degree, a misfit in a family of high achievers.

The medical evidence has been reviewed by Dr Richard Shepherd, forensic pathologist at St George's Medical School. The fact that the deep tissue injuries were so extensive did not in his view indicate that the wound had been inflicted with great force. The skin presents the greatest resistance to a penetrating injury and, once the skin has been perforated, a sharp instrument cuts freely into the soft tissues. The chisel was a very heavy one and it could gather great momentum if it were thrown. The evidence did not indicate that it had been stabbed in rather than being flicked across[3].

Everleigh was buried in Reigate cemetery beside his younger sister Lilian and this was the last time that the family plot was opened. To have the parents buried there would undoubtedly have rekindled old and unhappy memories. Everleigh's death was never mentioned in the family again and all family correspondence of that period has been destroyed.

Mary and John Langdon-Down had lost their first-born daughter and then their first-born son, heart-breaking tragedies which could have destroyed a couple with less strength of character or faith. They survived with their beliefs intact and their mutual affection strengthened. They never lost their stability nor their deep-rooted religious confidence. Incidentally a blood transfusion could have saved their son but this was, as yet, unavailable.

References

1 *Surrey Comet*. 11 August, 1883.
2 Death notice, *Surrey Comet*. 11 August, 1883.
3 Shepherd R. Personal communication, 1996.

Chapter 14

Down's Syndrome

Langdon Down's first objective was achieved when the learning disabled were separated from the insane and, in Earlswood, he moved on to try to divide residents according to their learning ability. The hope was that, by matching like with like, progress would be accelerated. In addition, he tried to break down the large number of patients into diagnostic groups. Langdon Down was greatly influenced by John Conolly, his mentor from early years. Conolly had a long-standing interest in ethnology and cranial differences between ethnic groups and his influence will be discussed later (Chapter 18).

The flattening of the back of the head, which is characteristic of Down's syndrome, was something which Langdon Down had observed at an early stage. Although his 'Ethnic Classification' does not mention the foreshortening of the head with a flattened back, his first Lettsomian Lecture draws attention to the ill-developed posterior part of the cranium. When he first went to Earlswood there was already a medical admission form which had been drawn up to comply with the requirements of the Lunacy Act. The form had been introduced in 1856 and required measurements of the skull's circumference, the distance between the root of the nose and the occipital prominence at the back of the head and the width of the forehead. The special apparatus, described as a measuring jack which was employed in Earlswood for these measurements, is preserved in the Royal Earlswood museum. It was manufactured by the Cambridge Instrument Company and essentially consisted of a wooden frame with calibrated measuring rods which were shortened or lengthened to make the measurements. Using the apparatus, the proportions of the head could be compared in a variety of different patients; the characteristic shape seen in Down's syndrome could be clearly identified. It was the facial characteristics, however, which particularly attracted his attention. He was later to lose faith in ethnology and, in Normansfield, no head measurements were recorded.

In his paper in the *Lancet* in 1862[1], written while at Earlswood, he published his observations on the condition of the mouth. He measured the palate and observed the condition of the tongue and teeth. A high arched palate was a frequent finding, but of greater interest was what he said about the tongue. Out of 200 cases examined he noted a special finding in 16; in these he reported that the tongue presented a sodden appearance and exhibited deep transverse fissures on its upper surface. He considered that patients with these findings had a marked physiological and psychological resemblance to each other, so much so that they might readily be taken as members of the same family. Presumably these were residents with Down's syndrome who showed a tongue abnormality which is common in the condition. In the 1866 *London Hospital Reports* Langdon Down published a paper entitled 'Observations on an Ethnic Classification of Idiots'[2]. The subject of the paper was to try and find a way of classifying the feeble minded, by arranging them within various ethnic standards. He drew his case material from Earlswood patients – whom he had painstakingly photographed in 1862 and 1865 – and from patients he had seen in the outpatients department at the London Hospital.

He kept his own notebooks and studied all the details carefully. It was from his notebooks, measurements and photographs that he came to distinguish a group of patients that he described as 'Mongolian'. Looking at his surviving photographs only about 5% appear to show typical appearances of Down's syndrome but he may have been working on the basis that every resident belonged to one of the ethnic groups and so may have decided that there was a hint of Mongolism in some whose appearance was not completely characteristic. His successor, Dr Grabham, was pressed by the Board of Earlswood to continue with Langdon Down's project of photographing the patients, but said that his workload made this impossible and, at that time, it was agreed to try and engage a professional photographer for the purpose[3]. This plan was approved in principle, but not all subsequent patients had photographs taken.

In his seminal paper on 'The Ethnic Classification of Idiots' Langdon Down began by stating that there are, of course, numerous representatives of the great Caucasian family. This important preamble has largely been overlooked by commentators on his work. His clear implication was that the greatest number of his patients were Caucasian in appearance and this reflects the common experience, that patients with learning disability do not have any special facial or other characteristics which separate them from the main stream of their peer group. He describes three other groups in addition to Mongolian, the first made up of those who have 'Ethiopian' characteristics – with prominent eyes, puffy lips, a receding chin and woolly hair – resembling white Negroes. Another group he described as 'Malayan' in appearance and a third as 'Aztec'. Those with Aztec characteristics had shortened foreheads, prominent cheeks, deep-set eyes and a rather aquiline nose and may have suffered from the Cornelia de Lange type of microcephaly, in which the patient suffers from severe disability, related to a marked degree of reduction in the size of the cranium, together with a characteristic facial appearance, with heavy eyebrows and other malformations. There are, however, no typical cases among the photographs that have survived.

His most important observation related to the group who he described as 'Mongolian'. In his view the resemblance between affected patients was so marked that, when placed side by side, it was difficult to believe they were not the children of the same parents. He went on to describe a typical child. He said:

> ...the hair is not black as in the real Mongol, but a brownish colour, straight and scanty. The face is flat and broad, and destitute of prominence. The cheeks are rounded and extended laterally. The eyes are obliquely placed, and the internal canthi more than normally distant from one another. The palpebral fissure is very narrow. The forehead is wrinkled transversely from the constant assistance from which the levators help the palpebrum to rise from the occipito-frontalis muscle and the opening of eyes. The lips are large and thick with transverse fissures. The tongue is long, thick and much roughened. The nose is small. The skin has a slight dirty yellowish tinge, and is deficient in elasticity, being of the appearance of being too large for the body. The boy's aspect is such that it is difficult to realize he is the child of Europeans, but so frequently are these characters presented that there can be no doubt that these ethnic features are the result of degeneration.
>
> The Mongolian type of idiocy occurs in more than 10% of the cases which are presented to me. They are always congenitally based and never result from accidents after uterine life. They are for the most part instances of degeneracy from tuberculosis in the parents...They have considerable power of imitation, even bordering on being mimics. They are humorous and a lively sense of the ridiculous often colours their mimicry. This faculty of imitation may be cultivated to a great extent, and a practical direction given to the results obtained. They are usually able to speak: speech is thick and indistinct but may be improved greatly by a well directed scheme of tongue gymnastics. The coordinating faculty is abnormal but not so defective that they can not be greatly strengthened. By systematic training considerable manipulative power may be obtained. The circulation is feeble, and however much advance is made intellectually in the summer, some amount of retrogression may be expected in the winter[2].

He did not specifically identify congenital heart disease as a problem, although his student lectures from Dr Herbert Davies at the London Hospital must have given him a good grounding in cardiac examination. The fact that effective cardiac surgery did not emerge for almost a century after his description made the differential diagnosis of congenital heart disease an academic matter. He was aware of the problem and frequently described patients as having a feeble circulation. There was no clinical incentive to proceed further in distinguishing specific details of cardiac abnormality, as nothing could be done for even the simplest of defects at that time. Additionally, patients were not admitted to Earlswood until the age of seven. In the days before diuretics, antibiotics and, of course, surgery, the children with Down's syndrome who had congenital heart disease had a very poor prognosis and there were probably few survivors.

He identified a seasonal change in active development, suggesting that some of his Mongolian patients had associated thyroid deficiency, a known complication of Down's syndrome. Hypothyroid patients do not tolerate the cold. Perhaps, having seen hypothyroidism develop in some of his patients, he may have exaggerated the effect it produced, but he must have noted the clinical picture of thyroid deficiency for him to remark on the problem of winter slowdown.

His thinking with regard to the significance of the ethnic classification requires explanation. He stated that the the departure of certain patients from the physical characteristics of their own race, and their assumption of the characteristics of others, is evidence of favour of unity of the human species. The differences between races were, in his view, not specific, but represented a variation in the natural spectrum of development. His philosophical views will be discussed later (Chapter 18). The point he wished to make was that, as oriental looking children could be born to European parents, both must come from the same stock rather than be separately descended from different animal species. Fanciful derivation of Caucasians from chimpanzee stock, Mongolians from orang-utans and Negroes from the gorilla emerged after his death. Crookshank was one of those who followed this line and, in 1924, he published a book *The Mongol in our Midst*[4], in which photographs of gorillas, chimpanzees and orang-utans were pictured side by side with their alleged human descendants. Crookshank made great play of the fact that the single transverse skin crease seen in the palm of the Mongolian child was seen only in the orang-utan. He also drew a parallel between the posture of both species. His book represented a perversion of John Langdon Down's views, although he did use the Langdon Down name, referring to Reginald's findings on the palmar crease.

After his initial identification of the specific picture of the Mongolian idiot, Langdon Down moved away from the concept of degenerative genetic inheritance leading to physical characteristics appropriate to another racial stock. Speaking in a discussion in 1867 on a paper by Richardson, entitled *Physical Disease from Mental Strain*, Langdon Down said that he had abandoned his belief in phrenology after 10 years of study and had rejected the view that a

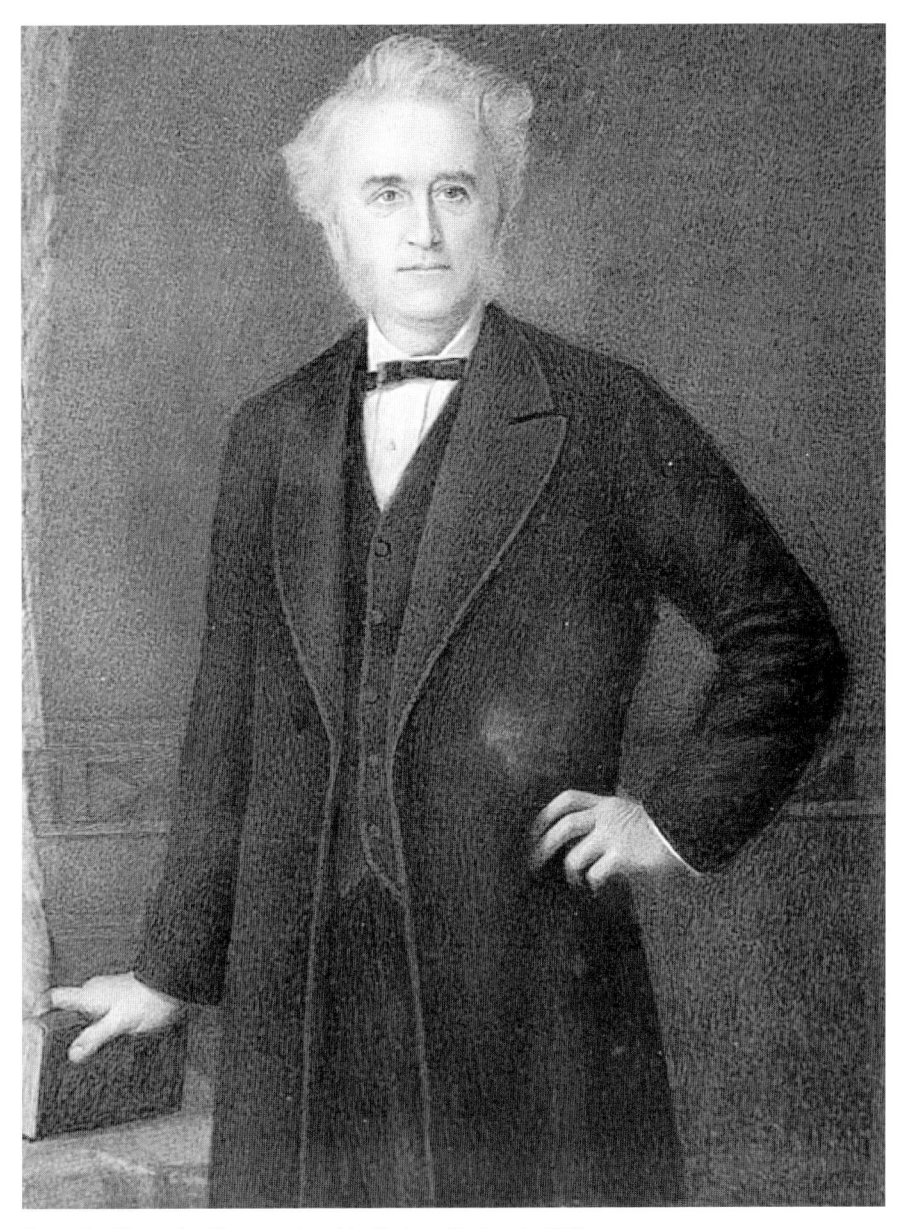

Portrait of Langdon Down, painted by Sydney Hodges in 1883.

person's character and intelligence could be deduced from the outer appearance and shape of his skull[5].

When Langdon Down was invited to write the section on Idiocy in Quain's *Dictionary of Medicine* in 1882, he made no mention of racial characteristics as being important in the diagnosis. His Mongolian group were simply listed as 'strumous'. He had, for practical purposes, abandoned the ethnic concept of there being racial implications in the physical appearance of these idiots he classified as Mongolian[6].

Mongolian idiots: Langdon Down's impact

The fact that not all those affected by learning disability should be viewed in the same light and that there were specific recognizable characteristics in some sub-groups was a totally new concept. It was quite remarkable that, before Langdon Down's description, nobody had separated out the Mongolian type from other forms of handicap. One example of this was the great Charles West, the founding father of the Great Ormond Street Hospital for Sick Children. He wrote a paper in 1860 entitled 'The Mental Peculiarities and the Mental Disorders of Childhood'[7] in which no mention was made of the specific characteristics of Down's syndrome. Griesinger, referred to with approval by Langdon Down in his first Lettsomian Lecture, had described microcephalic and Aztec types and also the premature fusion of the bony components of the skull, but made no reference to either Mongolian or Kalmuk idiots[8]. It is just possible that Edouard Séguin, in his book on *Idiocy and its Treatment by the Physiological Method*[9] includes in fact a brief description of what is now called 'Down's syndrome'. Having discussed cretinism and goitre he goes on to say in relation to what he calls 'furfuraceous cretinism' that the affected subjects showed 'milk-white rosy and peeling skin, with the shortcoming of all the integuments, which give an unfinished aspect to the truncated fingers and nose, with cracked lips and tongue, and with red ectropic conjunctiva coming out to supply the curtailed skin at the margins of the lids'. Séguin's description however lacks the clarity of Down's and it seems indisputable that Langdon Down should continue to take precedence in the matter of eponymity.

Séguin was aware of the need to subdivide the learning disabled into functional categories but was of the opinion that 'our incomplete studies do not permit actual classification; but it is better to leave things by themselves than to force them into classes which have their foundation only on paper'[9]. Likewise Duncan and Willard in their *Manual for the Classification, Training and Education of the Feeble Minded, Imbecile and Idiotic* in 1866 go no further than a functional description of the grades of handicap; clinical sub-groups are not identified[10].

Arthur Mitchell was a contemporary who also took up the question of classification of the physical characteristics of patients with learning disability. He wrote in the *Edinburgh Medical Journal*:

> There are however, certain forms of idiocy which patients properly classed under traumatic idiocy would never exhibit. One of these,

for instance, which is detached from the other forms of idiocy by lines as clear as those which separate mania from melancholia has invariably had intrauterine origin and there is good reason to believe that the abnormalities which it presents dates from the early months of pregnancy. A case of this kind could not be classed as one of traumatic idiocy, in the meaning at least that we give to that term[11].

Mitchell was Commissioner in Lunacy with responsibility for visiting all the institutions in Scotland. In association with Robert Fraser, but not until 1876, he published a detailed report on what he described as 'Kalmuc idiocy', referring to the critical facial characteristics which he described as being typical of the Kalmuc race. He also described the detailed appearance and the autopsy findings in a patient called Elizabeth Meldrum and gave an account of 62 patients he had seen in the course of his work. Mitchell noted that such patients were rarely seen in the Scottish Asylums and 60 of his 62 observed cases lived at home, he pointed out in particular their short life span[11]. He made no reference to Langdon Down's 1866 paper, despite the fact that he should have seen it at the time of its second publication in 1867, for it was republished in the very same journal that accepted his paper[12]. He clearly should not have overlooked Down's paper; did he simply choose to ignore it? Mitchell and Fraser must, however, be given credit for publishing the first lithograph of an affected young man, taken from a photograph of a patient 'the name of whom I have omitted to preserve'. Although Langdon Down had taken a large number of photographs, he never published any engravings of them.

The timing of Mitchell's publication probably explains Langdon Down's decision to reprint his early papers together with his Lettsomian Lectures (see Chapter 17). The volume of reprinted articles includes his 1866 paper on the Ethnic Classification, now in fact published for the third time. Presumably this was a reminder to the medical profession of his prior contribution to the knowledge of the subject. There was no other good reason for even reprinting the Lettsomian Lectures, as these had already been reported at length in the *BMJ* in 1887[13]. The first and third lectures had also been published almost verbatim in the *Medical Press and Circular*. The information they contained had been widely diffused. Langdon Down effectively established his prior right to the authorship of the first description of a previously unrecognized condition and, from then on the term 'Mongolian idiocy' was commonly used as a descriptive term. The alternative designation of 'Kalmuc idiocy' never achieved popular consent and support in medical circles for its use never became widespread.

It took time for the new idea to filter through to the medical profession. Charles West's paper in the *Medical Gazette* has been referred to and, in addition, West's 1868 textbook on diseases of children does not refer to Mongolian idiots[14]. This may, however, have been a simple consequence of the infrequency of admission of Down's syndrome patients to his unit in the Great Ormond Street Hospital for Sick Children at that time. Other authors however took up the description of Mongolian idiocy and, in 1879, Tanner and Meadows quoted Down's description of the Ethnic Classification of Idiocy[15]. So did Goodhart in his textbook *The Diseases of Children*[16]. In this he also showed interest in Down's observations on developmental idiocy, a disorder in which children developed normally to a certain point and then became imbecile, with no further brain development, sometimes as a result of a fit or of some postulated impaired nutrition. By 1891 in the US the *Encyclopedia of the Diseases of Children*, edited by Keating and Young, published a contribution by Edward Brush, in which he quoted Down's description of the classification of the idiots at great length[17].

Two major reviews on learning disability appeared in 1903 and 1909. Tredgold wrote extensively in the *Practitioner* on all aspects of learning disability, including a classification. He identifies Mongolian idiots, but makes no reference to Langdon Down[18]. Shuttleworth, writing in the *BMJ* in 1909 about Mongolian idiocy, did give credit to Langdon Down for his observations, although he disagreed with Langdon Down's theory of ethnic regression[19].

Questions have been raised as to why this clearly identified and easily recognized condition had not been studied before Langdon Down drew attention to it. There were a number of reasons for this. To begin with, infant mortality was extremely high. At the time up to one quarter of all infants died in their first year of life. When healthy children had a high mortality, children affected by the condition described by Down could be expected to die in great numbers and to have poor survival rates. Secondly, in the 1850s only about half the women in England reached the age of 35, beyond which the incidence of Down's syndrome increases[20]. The pool of older mothers who were more at risk of having affected children was therefore notably smaller. These figures were given in a letter to the *Lancet* by Richards, who estimated that in Shakespeare's time there were no more than 100 Down's syndrome patients in the whole of England[20]. The art galleries of Europe had been scoured for portraits of children with Down's syndrome from earlier ages. Dr Tom Cone from Boston suggested in the *Lancet* in 1968 that the first pictorial representation was in a painting by Mantegna circa 1500[21]. Another possibility is that the Mongolian or Down's syndrome patients lived in seclusion in the community and rarely reached the active teaching hospitals where most medical observations were made. They lived quietly and died young, almost unnoticed by the medical profession.

References

1. Down JL. On the condition of the mouth in infancy. *Lancet* 1862; **1**: 65–8.
2. Down JL. Observations on an Ethnic Classification of Idiots. *London Hospital Reports*. 1862; **3**: 259–62.
3. SRO/392/3/1/11. Surrey Record Office.
4. Crookshank FG. *The Mongol in our Midst*. London: Kegan Paul, Trench, Trubner and Co, 1924.
5. Down JL. Discussion. *J Ment Sc* 1868; **13**: 472.
6. Quain R, ed. *Dictionary of Medicine*. London: Longmans Green, 1882: 925.
7. West C. The mental peculiarities and mental disorders of childhood. *Med Times & Gazette* 1860: 134–7.
8. Griesinger W. *Mental Pathology and Therapeutics*. Translated: Robertson CL, Rutherford J. London: New Sydenham Society, 1867.
9. Séguin E. *Idiocy and its treatment by the physiological method*. Wood & Co, 1866.
10. Duncan PM, Willard AW. *Manual for the Classification, Training and Education of the Feeble Minded*. Longman Green, 1866.
11. Mitchell A, Fraser R. Kalmuc Idiocy. *J Ment Sc* 1876; **22**: 169–79.
12. Down JL. Ethnic classification of idiots. *J Ment Sc* 1867–8; **13**: 121–3.
13. *BMJ* 1887; **1**: 49–50, 149–51, 256–9.
14. West C. *Diseases of Infancy and Childhood*. London: Longman Green, 1868.
15. Tanner TH, Meadows A. *Diseases of Infancy and Childhood*. London: Renshaw, 1879.
16. Goodhart JF. *The Diseases of Children*. JA Churchill, 1888.
17. Keating JM, Young J, eds. *Encyclopedia of the Diseases of Children*. Pentland, 1891.
18. Tredgold AF. Amentia. *Practitioner* 1903; **2**: 354–82.
19. Shuttleworth GE. Clinical Lecture on Idiocy and Imbecility. *BMJ* 1886: 183–6.
20. Richards BW. Correspondence. *Lancet* 1968; **2**: 253.
21. Cone TE. Correspondence. *Lancet* 1968; **2**: 829.

Chapter 15

Reginald and Percival Langdon Down

Reginald was born in the family accomodation in Earlswood in 1866, the third of the Langdon Down children; his sister, Lilian, had died the year before. At the time his father was in the throes of a measles epidemic and was also finishing his 'Ethnic Classification', so Reginald probably saw very little of him in his early years. Percival was born in 1868, within a week of the Langdon Down's move to Normansfield; Everleigh was then age six and Reginald two. The room in which Percival was born became the Normansfield pharmacy in later years. There are, unfortunately, no surviving childhood photographs of either Reginald or Percival.

Schooldays

The Langdon Down boys were taken to a local preparatory school and travelled each day by pony and trap. Everleigh, the eldest, did not go to public school, but Reginald and Percival were sent at the age of nine to the preparatory school run by the Reverend Henry Tottenham, so from an early age they were away from home. They went on to Harrow at the age of 12 and, from then until they completed their University education, were only at home during holidays.

At school it was clear that Percival was closest to his mother. The schoolboy letters say nothing about any trauma from parental separation, but it was Percival who wrote regularly to 'My Dearest Mother'. If Reginald needed a new scarf, Percival was the one to write and ask for it; Percival also reported on how Reginald was progressing in school.

When at home the boys were very involved in the everyday life and activities, first in Earlswood and then Normansfield, particularly in the entertainments and theatre productions in which they frequently performed (see Chapter 12). Their parents lived life alongside the residents and their children did the same during school holidays. It is not therefore surprising that they were at ease when, eventually, they took over the running of Normansfield after the death of both their parents.

Coming of Age

There were two very big celebrations at Normansfield as each of the sons came of age. Everleigh was clearly not so highly regarded; there was no public celebration of his coming of age in the year before he died. He was, it seems, something of a nineteenth century dropout. In 1887 Reginald's coming of age coincided with the celebrations of Queen Victoria's Jubilee. The entire staff were lavishly entertained but, before the festivities, a summer fair was held for the children who lived in Normansfield. They had a Punch and Judy show, performing dogs, clowns and games until dusk, and then the grounds were lit up in a brilliant display of fairy lights[1].

The staff were entertained to supper in the children's assembly hall and there was dancing to the music of the Normansfield orchestra until midnight. Reginald received a handsome gold watch from his parents, to which was added a heavy gold chain, a gift from other relatives; the staff presented him with a travelling bag. On the same occasion Walter Lee, the head coachman, received a silver cup in celebration of 21 years' service.

Percival's coming of age party in 1889 was spread over two days; on the first day 600 guests were invited and, on the second, 400. Ten thousand fairy lamps had been hung in the grounds by the Brock Company, who had been responsible for the illuminations at Crystal Palace. All the company were in evening dress and danced to the music of the Anglo-Hungarian Band. The Brock Company closed the evening with a magnificent firework display, the set pieces including the monogram of Percival Langdon Down. Percival too, got his gold watch and chain. The chain probably came from Sarah and Philip Crellin – his uncle and aunt – who had befriended his father as a medical student and in his first year in Earlswood. The staff presented Percival with a diamond stud and pin; Mr Hibbs, the leader of the Normansfield orchestra, made the presentation and said in his speech that he hoped Percival would follow in the footsteps of his worthy father. For London guests a special train had been arranged, leaving Hampton Wick Station at 12.40 am. On this occasion there were two staff presentations, one to William Briggs, who had been in service for 21 years as an attendant, and a second to Caroline, his wife[2].

Travel

The Langdon Down family, once the boys were older, were able to travel widely. They visited Paris, Italy and Germany and made a summer trip to Norway. The longest family trip was undertaken in 1887, when Langdon Down travelled to Canada and the US to attend the World Medical Congress in New York. The family travelled on the Cunarder SS *Servia* from Liverpool on 27th August and docked in New York on 5th September. Transatlantic vessels sailing from Liverpool to New York at that time put in to Queenstown, now Cobh, on the southwest coast of Ireland. The return journey began on 1st October and the family disembarked in

Liverpool on 8th October. They returned to London by train. After attending the New York conference, where Langdon Down presented a re-statement of his findings of Down's syndrome, they travelled to Montreal and then took a tour of the Niagara Falls. It must have been a most interesting journey for Reginald and Percival, then aged 21 and 19.

Normansfield Through the Generations

As boys, Reginald and Percival were introduced to a relative life of luxury and both relished the lifestyle to which their father's wealth had introduced them. When Reginald moved into Normansfield after his mother's death in 1901, he set about furnishing it in grand style, with an emphasis on Chinese porcelain and antique furniture. Number 81 Harley Street remained in the family but neither son became actively involved in the development of the consulting practice and the property was sold in 1901.

Reginald married Jane Jarvey Cleveland, a ward sister at the London Hospital, in 1895. His daughter, Elspie, grew up to become an accomplished artist and taught arts and crafts in Normansfield. Three weaving looms which she used were still in Normansfield when it was taken over by the National Health Service in 1951. Reginald's other daughter, Stella, was to become Lady Brain, having married Dr Russell Brain. Reginald and Jane had one son, John, who was ultimately diagnosed – ironically – as having Down's syndrome. John lived to the ripe old age of 65. He was a very lovable person and, once it was realized that he could not make good progress at the local school, was absorbed into the Normansfield training programme. Numeracy remained a problem for him throughout his life, although he had other well-developed skills and was a good billiard player. When the National Health Service took over the running of Normansfield in 1951, John remained on as a private patient. He walked out with his carer, enjoyed music and his health remained good until a lingering infection affected him in his last year. Reginald's wife, Jane, died in 1917, having been ill for some time. After being a widower for five years he then married Ruth Turnbull and they had one son, Tony, who has remained to the fore in the Friends of Normansfield, a registered charity devoted to the interests of people with learning difficulties.

Percival married Mouche, the second daughter of James Bigwood, MP of Twickenham. He was very much in the mould of his father, giving his time to patient care and public affairs. He was Chairman of Teddington Urban Council, the lock staff committee of the Thames Conservancy, Richmond Bridge Commissioners and the Thames Valley Councils Association. When Mary Langdon Down died in 1901, Reginald and his wife Jane administered Normansfield while Percival maintained the clinical service. When Reginald's wife died,

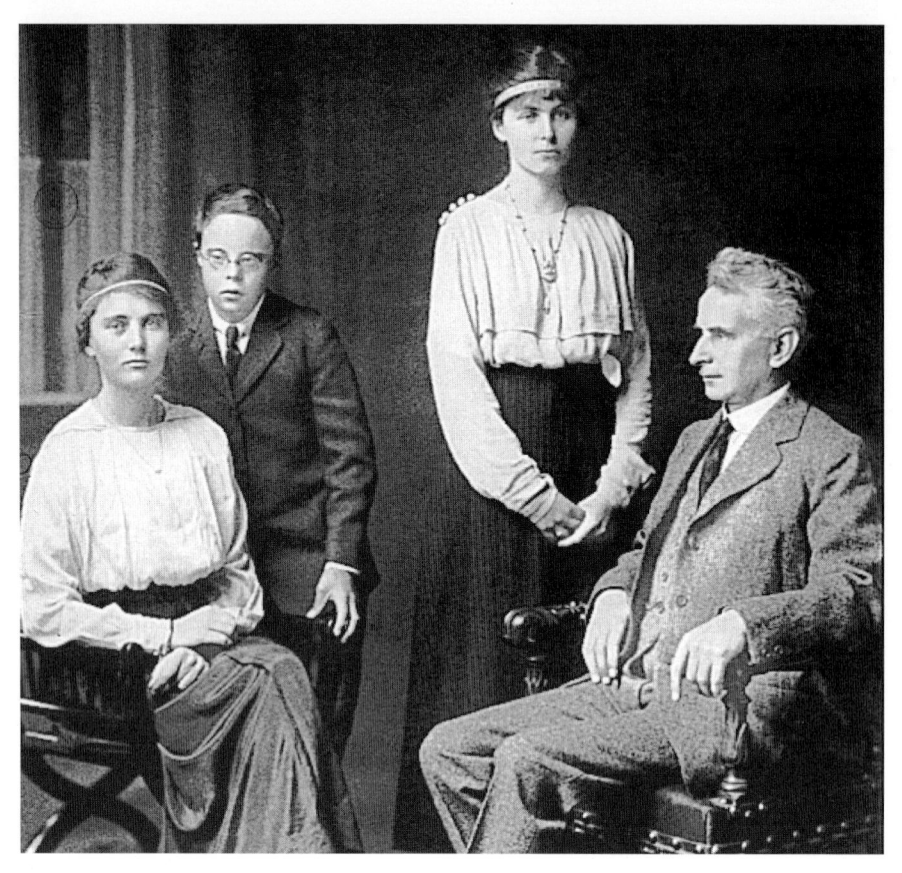

Dr Reginald Langdon Down with his daughters Stella and Elspie. Stella married Russell Brain and became Lady Brain. Elspie was an artist. The only son was John, who had Down's syndrome.

Percival's wife stepped in to fill the breach, which she continued to do even after Percival's death in 1925, when Normansfield became a limited company.

The Second World War crippled Normansfield as a private institution. It had survived undamaged in German bombing raids, but was in financial straits and passed to the National Health Service in 1951. The Langdon Down link continued and Dr Norman Langdon Down remained as superintendent until his retirement in 1970. Lady Stella Brain, Reginald's daughter, who had assisted with the management of the private institution, retained a voluntary connection until she died in 1991. For over a century three generations of medical Langdon Downs had supervised the Institution and, throughout that long period, it retained the reputation of a fine and well-managed institution. This unfortunately came to an end in 1974 when, under National Health Service management, the conditions in Normansfield provoked an official enquiry and, subsequently, a critical report[3].

Down's Syndrome Research

Following his father's description and identification of Down's syndrome, Reginald made a further contribution to the subject in 1905, when he presented 14 cases of Down's syndrome at the autumn meeting of the South Eastern Division of the Medical Psychological Society. The meeting was held at Normansfield and was subsequently reported in the *Journal of Mental Science* in January 1906[4].

Of the 14 Down's syndrome patients he presented, nine were adults; from the records it would appear that five of the latter were his father's patients, still in residence in Normansfield. His oldest patient at that time was 56; she had in fact been the first Down's syndrome patient admitted to Normansfield by his father at the age of 19. The average age of his adult patients was 35 years; they were in general short, around five feet in height and their head circumferences on average were 20.75 inches, compared with the normal adult average of 22.5 inches. He produced diagrams to show the characteristic shape of the head, with the reduced front to back diameter. In general the adult head size was the equivalent of that of a boy aged 12 years. The proportion of Down's syndrome patients in Normansfield at that time was 9.7%, corresponding closely with the incidence identified by his father in Earlswood. He had noted that the mortality among his 'Mongolian' patients was higher than that observed among other learning disabled patients.

Reginald noted that the affected children were often the last of a large family and, indeed, one was the youngest of 15; also 60% of families had a history of tuberculosis. He felt that the debility of the mother during pregnancy was an important factor and had been concerned about a patient from Holland whose mother had been placed on a restricted diet during the last five months of her pregnancy; he felt that this may have resulted in the condition of the child. His father would not have approved of this deduction, having decided in his own mind that the underlying flaw in the Mongolian idiot had its origin at the very moment of conception. He would have approved even less of Reginald's suggestion, on the same occasion, that Down's syndrome might be due to a reversion to a type more backward than primitive man. This later fuelled the fires of degenerationism (Chapter 14). An interesting contribution to this discussion came from Dr Fell, who had seen numerous cases in Darenth Asylum, where 5% of the patients were identified as Mongolian. His specific observation was that many of them suffered from congenital heart disease.

In the scientific sense Reginald's main contribution to medical science was the identification of the abnormal palmar crease in Down's syndrome. Contributing to a discussion on a paper by Dr Shuttleworth in 1909 he said:

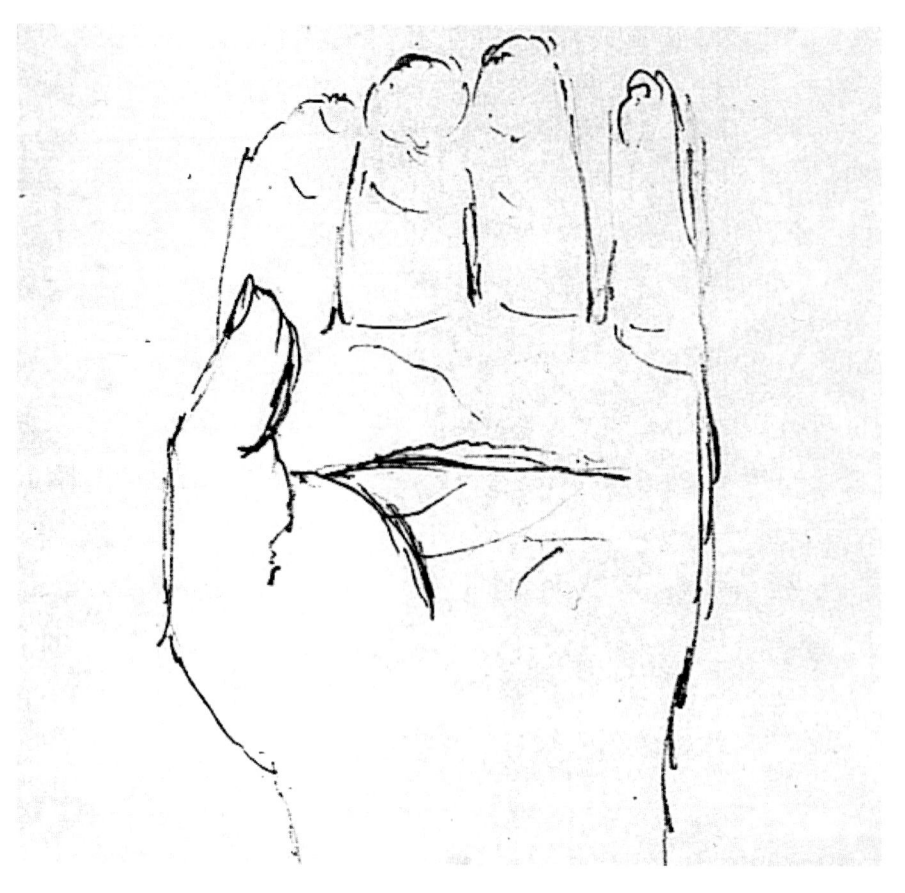

Reginald Langdon Down was the first to describe the pattern of creases in the palm in Down's syndrome patients. He drew this sketch in 1908.

...showed hand prints of a number of such cases compared with a normal hand print. These showed a marked shortening of the metacarpal bones and the phalanges, and the extreme suppleness of the joints was indicated by the superior ease with which the impress of the centre of the palm was obtained. In addition to the abnormality of the bony structures, these prints showed that the bones of the palm differed from the normal in their extreme irregularity, and the tendency of the principal fold-lines to be two in number only, instead of three as was most commonly the case[5].

Reginald's sketch of the palm is in the family papers, dated 1908.
 Reginald confirmed his father's previous estimate of the Mongolian children forming 10% of, as he described it, 'the imbecile group'. He drew attention to the fact that the prognosis for reaching adult life was poor and that they frequently died from tuberculosis or other pulmonary disease. It is tempting to speculate

that his observation on the palm had also been the result of an input from his father. John Langdon Down published nothing after 1887 and was criticized for this in his own time and subsequently.

Both Reginald and Percival, who qualified in medicine in 1892 and 1893 respectively, worked effectively as his assistants, having gone quickly into the field of learning disability. Their only training was the training their father had given them. He may in consequence, deserve to share the credit for Reginald's observations. There was, as it were, a Langdon Down school of study on learning disability. Unfortunately, neither Reginald or Percival published any medical papers. Reginald's observations on the hand were simply included in a *BMJ* report of the discussion on a major paper by George Shuttleworth, Honorary Consulting Physician at the Royal Albert Asylum in Lancaster.

Reginald also noted that Mongolian children appeared in families after a long interval of non-childbearing. He was on the threshold of identifying the age-specific increase in the frequency of Down's syndrome, related to maternal ageing. He did not, however, make the final leap and it was not until the next century that this issue was clarified. Reginald also noted that the shortening of the facial bones resulted in narrowing of the nasal passages. The clinical importance of this factor in increasing the susceptibility to upper respiratory infection is well-known.

Reginald's Other Medical Interests

As a medical trainee, he had shown promise and Stephen Mackenzie, his medical mentor in the London Hospital, considered his work to be very good and described him as 'exceedingly able'. When he completed his house appointment Mackenzie promised him full support in the future. After Reginald qualified, he may have started off with the intention of becoming a hospital consultant. He passed the examination for membership of the Royal College of Physicians in 1894, two years after graduating at the London Hospital and, on completion of his House Officer appointment, put his foot on the first rung of the academic ladder by becoming a demonstrator in anatomy in the London Hospital Medical School. He may then simply have been sucked in to the vortex of activity in Normansfield; in addition Normansfield was generating a large income which made it unnecessary for him to establish his own independent share of medical practice.

Reginald had an interest in eugenics and went against the stream of professional opinion in advocating sterilization on eugenic grounds, at least in some cases. His proposal was voted down at the Conference on Mental Welfare in 1930 and, amongst those who opposed it, was Tredgold, one of the leading experts on handicap[6].

He was actively interested in medical photography, having no doubt observed his father's involvement and, in 1916, reviewed his father's photographs. He then set about completing a comprehensive photographic survey of the contemporary Normansfield residents – his 180 paired front and side views are now in the London Metropolitan Records Office. Reginald was President of the Section of Psychiatry of the Royal Society of Medicine; he presented an address on the Report of the Royal Commission on Lunacy. He clearly had the intellectual endowment to make further contributions to medical science, but the management of Normansfield took him out of the academic stream.

Percival's medical contribution

In 1895 both Reginald and Percival were added to the Commissioner's Licence for Normansfield and became increasingly involved. When their father died in 1896, they took over responsibility for the medical administration, while their widowed mother continued to organize the running of the establishment. Percival, who had qualified within a year, rather than two, of his older brother was clearly very bright, but did not take any higher qualifications. He appears to have been a people's person and his forte was in the daily care of the patients. He died in 1925 and his

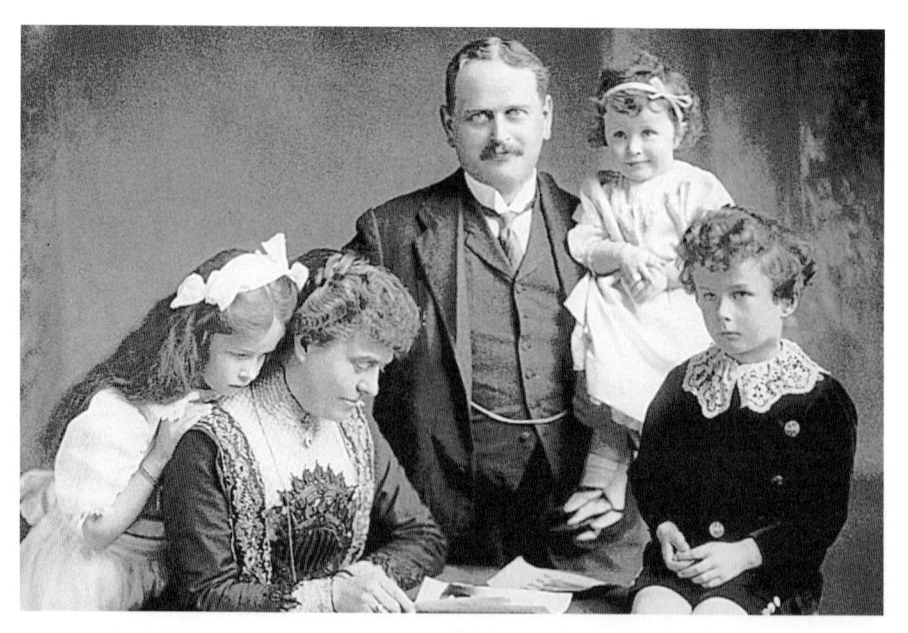

Dr Percival Langdon Down with his wife and children. His son Norman, was to be the last Langdon Down superintendent of Normansfield, ending a family connection that had lasted for 102 years. The elder daughter, Molly, was also a doctor and worked in Normansfield.

local obituary described him as a gifted, earnest, self-sacrificing man whose service to others would be difficult to overestimate. 'By nature he was a modest, retiring gentleman. A quiet placidity was his strength and the inspiration of a widespread public confidence and admiration'[7].

The interest in medicine was handed down in his family and, in due course, his son Norman qualified in medicine, took his specialist qualification in psychiatry and later became Medical Superintendent of Normansfield. His daughter Molly also took up psychiatry and worked in Normansfield for over a decade. She was the only Langdon Down to make a further contribution to the medical literature and, in 1929, was the main author of a paper with Russell Brain on how epileptic attacks were distributed around the clock and related to special times of day or night in individual cases[8].

An Unfortunate Resignation

In the *Medical Directory* for 1929 Reginald Langdon Down is listed as a Member of the Royal College of Physicians of London but, in 1930, this higher qualification is no longer listed. His *Lancet* obituary[9] in fact refers to his having resigned the membership when Normansfield became a Limited Company, which it did in 1926.

Membership of the Royal College of Physicians is hard-earned. To resign it is almost unknown and he can hardly have resigned willingly. In 1922 there was a great deal of discussion in the College concerning medical men who owned, or had a proprietary interest in, institutions from which they benefited by way of profit, from institutional budget balance as well as from professional fees. A resolution was passed on 25th October, 1888 which said: 'It is undesirable that any Fellow or Member of the College should be officially connected with any company having for its object the treatment of disease for profit'[10]. This was a resolution of the College and not a binding bye-law. John Langdon Down had never been at risk of censure in this connection as his wife, Mary, was the registered proprietor of Normansfield. His role was that of Medical Superintendent and the Normansfield accounts were kept separate from his practice accounts. It was not until the year before he died that John Langdon Down's name was entered as a partner with that of his wife in the ownership of Normansfield.

The bye-law of 1888 did not become a matter of dispute until 1922 when the College Comitia, its governing body, set out that 'it was undesirable that any Fellow or Member of the College should have any financial interest in any company or institution, having for its object the treatment of disease for profit, other than the receipt by him from such company or institution of a reasonable fixed salary or fees on an adequate scale for such services as he might render to such company or institution in his capacity of medical practitioner'[10]. The problem for Reginald was that, in 1926, Normansfield was incorporated as a limited company and, as a shareholder, he found himself to be in breach of the College resolution.

No relevant correspondence has been preserved by the College and there is no official letter from the College in Reginald Langdon Down's papers (in the London Metropolitan Records Office). It may be that he received a private warning from the President or Registrar. In any event he resigned his Membership of the Royal College. There would appear to be no doubt that his resignation was based on a matter of principle. His obituary of 4th June, 1955 states: 'Later, when Normansfield became a limited company, he insisted on resigning his MRCP, though to the regret of his colleagues'[9].

References

1 *Surrey Comet*. 6 July 1887.
2 *Kingston and Surbiton News*. 6 July, 1889.
3 London Metropolitan Records Office. LMRO;H29/NF/F/8/1–9.
4 *J Men Sc* 1906; **62**: 187–90.
5 Report. *BMJ* 1909; **2**: 665.
6 Conference on Mental Welfare: Report. *BMJ* 1930; **2**: 159–60.
7 Obituary. *Surrey Comet*. 22 August, 1925.
8 Langdon Down M, Brain R. Time of day in relation to convulsions in epilepsy. *Lancet* 1929; **2**: 1028–30.
9 Obituary. *Lancet* 1955: **1**; 1279–80.
10 Report from the Censor's Board, Royal College of Physicians. 28 April, 1922. Resolution of 25 October, 1888.

Chapter 16

Down's Syndrome Patients in Normansfield

Langdon Down recognized that the complex grouping of physical characteristics which he had noted must be due to an adverse influence affecting the foetus in the earliest stages of development, although the underlying chromosomal abnormality was not recognized for almost a century after his description. The histories of his Earlswood families made it clear that there was a very high incidence of tuberculosis among the parents of his 'Mongolian' children. He felt at first that with so specific a group there should be a single cause and, in his paper on idiocy and its relation to tuberculosis in the *Lancet* in 1867 went on to say:

> ...the subjects of this class assume the Mongolian type: while they present a marked similarity in external conformation they are characterized by the same mental and moral peculiarities; so that, given a case of the Mongolian type, we are often able to trace its origin to tuberculosis and to predicate the extent of response to training that may be expected, and the tendencies it will evince. Moreover, the knowledge that is gained by this racial character assists in laying down some specific rules as to food, medicine and general hygiene without which the mental development would be but small. The power of progress is usually much greater than one would judge by an ordinary inspection. Such cases are extremely susceptible to climatic changes, and the winter is for them a period of mental and physical developmental rest. In the spring they put forward increased imitative and receptive powers, which compensate to some extent the period of hibernation[1].

As previously noted, John Langdon Down went on from the particular to the general in this connection. Tuberculosis was not understood to be an infective disorder when Langdon Down wrote this paper. He simply saw it as an adverse antenatal influence and saw that, whatever was wrong, the effects were apparent from the earliest stages of foetal development. His concern was, in the main, with prognosis.

His paper clearly indicates that he was aware of the imitative powers of those children he had described in his first Lettsomian Lecture and he emphasized that the recognition of the antenatal origin of this special category patient was of great importance, especially when the parents attempted to attribute blame to an attendant physician or nurse. The characteristic appearances made it possible to say for certain that the condition was congenital in origin and that no form of malpractice or negligence could be attributed to the professional attendants. He also drew attention to the fact that 'these children do not have a long career, very few reaching adult life, being prone to succumb to serious illness and become phthisical like their ancestors'[1]. He says that recognition of this special group has a practical bearing because it brings into prominence a class which was formerly not considered, and that had not had the attention given to it which it merited.

Langdon Down made personal notes on his Earlswood patients; unfortunately, his notebooks have never been located. The clinical records in Earlswood followed the form required by legislation of 1845, as amended in 1853; every admission had to have a full examination of all systems and an entry had to be made for every patient suggesting the cause of the condition. Causes entered were largely speculative – insanity among relatives, an antecedent history of tuberculosis, alcoholism and extraneous events (such as heat stroke, convulsions, illness) and congenital abnormality (such as hydrocephalus) were listed. The form of the examination did not facilitate the listing of specific diagnoses such as 'Mongolian idiocy'. When Langdon Down began his independent work in his own institution in Normansfield his records became more specific and he entered more definite diagnoses; it is therefore possible to trace from the records what he learned about 'Mongolian idiocy' from 1868 onwards[2].

Individual Cases

His first Normansfield 'Mongolian' patient, Mary A, was admitted on May 12, 1868 at the age of 19. Mary A was one of the controversial patients who had been living with an Earlswood staff member in Redhill. She had been there for 12 months and was noted to have been under Dr Down's observation:

> She is of lymphatic temperament, has coarse skin, lips furrowed and a long tongue with enlarged papillae. Her circulation is feeble and she is very liable to chilblains. She menstruates regularly. Her other bodily functions are normal. She is imbecile in mind. She talks very much but with a little indistinctness. She is extremely obstinate, will not walk beyond the grounds and this obstinacy is most marked at the period antecedent to her catamenia. She can write a letter and play some tunes from memory on the piano. She is affectionate and when she is free from ill temper, is witty and cheerful. She nurses a doll which she

Down's Syndrome Patients in Normansfield

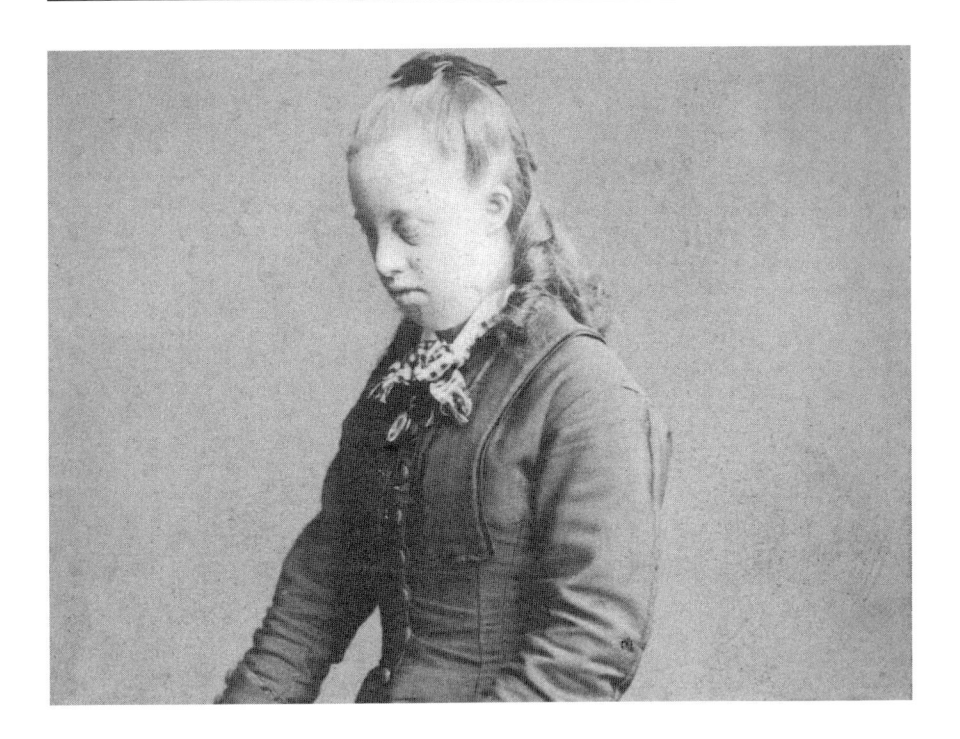

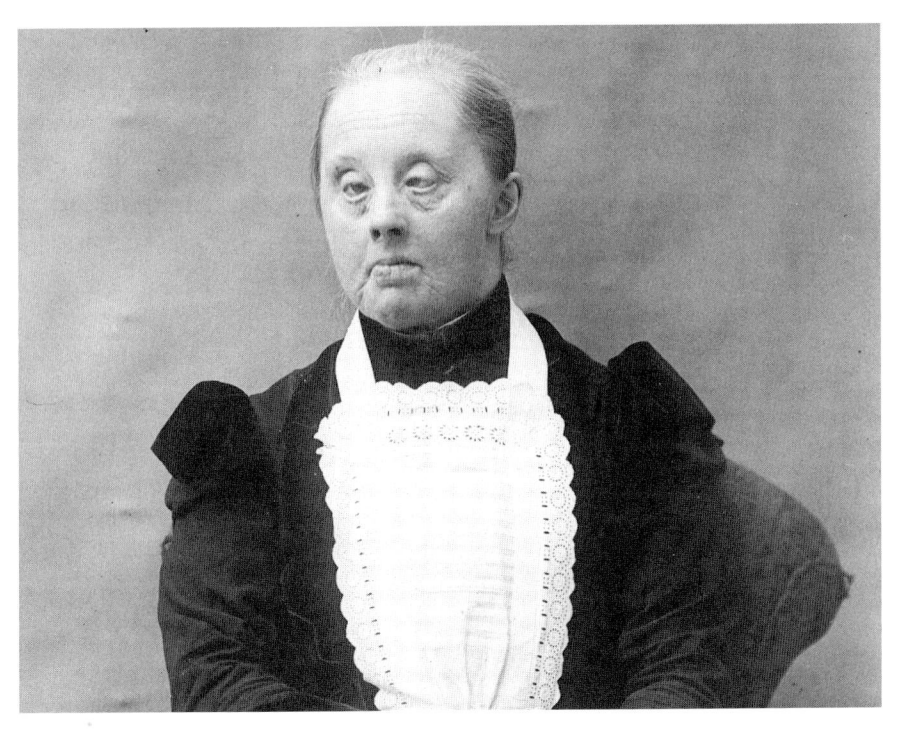

Mary A, the first Down's syndrome patient admitted to Normansfield, photographed when she was 19 and again when she was 55. She lived to the age of 58.

calls 'baby' and this baby is the one to whom all bad qualities are referred. Her mental peculiarities have existed from birth. Her father is healthy and of normal mental health. Her mother is highly nervous, delicate physically and mentally. She can partially dress herself only and can partially take care of her person. She is not epileptic. She has a slight tendency to lateral curvature of the spine and she stoops very much. She has converging strabismus and her voice is remarkably harsh[3]

Mary A lived an exceptionally long life. She had developed cardiac failure in her later years so presumably she had congenital heart disease, possibly a floppy mitral valve, the signs of which do not usually appear until late in life. She was also bedridden towards the end of her life and showed signs of dementia. The second patient was Cecilia Gertrude A who was admitted in 1868 at age 10. She was noted to have a disposition to purpura, a condition associated with low blood platelets and now known to be common in Down's syndrome. In December, 1869 she was taken ill with scarlet fever. One day later her temperature shot up to 106 degrees F and she had a seizure; within three hours her temperature had risen further to 107 degrees. Efforts were made to control her convulsions with bathing, which would be a perfectly standard procedure today. Neither aspirin nor paracetamol, which are now standard treatments for high temperature, had been discovered at that time and an effort was made to maintain cardiac function using sips of brandy and water. Her death was a great disappointment. Her progress notes had indicated that her behaviour was improving and that there were signs of increasing intelligence and encouraging progress.

Herbert H was admitted in July 1868 aged eight. It was recorded that there was a great disparity between the age of the father and mother, but the notes do not indicate whether it was the father or mother who was elderly. The main anxiety was that he had acquired the habit of swearing, having been allowed to mix with low people. In Normansfield he began to learn reading and writing and, when he was discharged, his behaviour was noted to have improved. Longevity, which was unexpected, was a feature of many of the patients, a tribute no doubt to the high staffing levels and good overall living conditions. Edward P, the fourth of Langdon Down's personal series of Mongolian patients, was admitted at the age of 11 in 1869. Next year he developed the rash of erythema nodosum, suggesting that he had contracted tuberculosis and, in the same year, he survived measles without complications. He was treated for bronchitis with a mustard poultice in 1874 and had inflammation of his legs in 1886. His convalescence was no doubt speeded up by the prescription of port wine. The dosage prescribed was conservative and he was given only one ounce three times daily. He lived to the age of 50.

Walter Abbot P was admitted in 1875 at the age of four. The parents were specially concerned in his case as he was given to masturbation; he was specially watched and discouraged and given chloral as a bedtime sedative. With these measures, the habit was broken and he was discharged two years later. Margaret E was 11 years old when she was admitted in 1874. Within a month she had contracted scarlet fever. Dr Gunther, a local general practitioner, was holding the fort as Langdon Down's locum for the evening but Langdon Down saw her himself at 1.30 am. He painted her tonsils with a strong solution of silver nitrate to try to control her infection at its source. This was repeated but, on the following day, Langdon Down was called to her at 3 am and again at 6 am. He found her improved but her condition deteriorated and Dr Gunther was called again to see her in consultation with Langdon Down; they tried stimulant therapy using half an ounce of brandy. Her temperature rose to 106 degrees and she was placed in a tepid bath after which she improved to the point of taking notice. She sank again and died after 15 minutes of unconsciousness. Scarlet fever, which could now be treated with penicillin was, at that time, frequently fatal, especially among handicapped children. Details of the other patients are set out in the table (see over). Of the 15 patients with Down's syndrome who died in Normansfield, two died of scarlet fever, one in 1870 and the other in the course of a mini epidemic in 1874. This was still a very virulent infection at the time. Five patients died of respiratory infection; in the absence of antibiotics, bronchitis and pneumonia had a very high mortality.

Of the five patients who lived beyond the age of 45, four had evidence of mental deterioration and may well have suffered from the early onset of Alzheimer's disease. One of these had cardiac failure and, despite the known incidence of congenital heart disease in Down's syndrome, this was one of the only two deaths from uncomplicated cardiac failure. The second death occurred in association with pneumonia. However, the deaths of nine patients below the age of 15 may have eliminated some of those patients who, if they had lived longer, might also have shown signs of cardiac complications. It was remarkable that only one patient died of tuberculosis. In this particular case the diagnosis was not definite. The low incidence of tuberculosis among the Normansfield patients may have been the result of cautious selection of healthy, non-infected attendants and also the nursery-style bedrooms, which meant that only small groups of residents were in close contact with each other.

The series of Down's syndrome patients in Normansfield illustrates the two perceptions of the role of the institution. On the one hand six of the patients might be regarded as almost permanent admissions, having remained resident for over 35 years. Only three

Langdon Down's personal patients with his syndrome[2]

Name	Age Admitted	Date Admitted	Outcome	Comment
Mary A	19	12.5.68	Died 1907, age 58	Cardiac failure, Alzheimer's
Cecelia GA	10	7.6.68	Died 31.1.70, age 12	Fatal scarlet fever
Herbert H	8	15.7.68	Discharged 10.10.68	Improved
Edward GP	11	1.5.69	Died 1908, age 50	
Laura M	7	5.4.69	Died 5.4.77, age 15	Tuberculosis: Query
Walter AP	4	4.11.75	Discharged 27.1.77	Masturbation cured
Margaret DE	11	14.4.74	Died 15.5.74, age 11	Fatal scarlet fever
Norah MT	12	23.4.74	Died 26.6.74, age 12	Acute Bronchitis
James DKW	5	10.1.77	Died 30.12.77, age 12	Bronchitis and Pneumonia
Norman MB	10	14.2.77	Died 12.1.12, age 45	Alzheimer's?
Thomas N	6	13.11.77	Died 1896, age 25	Cardiac failure
Margaret AW	4	11.3.80	Died 1885, age 9	Sudden death on holiday
George HW	6	27.3.80	Died 27.11.80, age 7	Laryngo bronchitis, croup
Cathy MS	9	28.3.82	Died 20.8.82, age 9	Bronchitis and pneumonia
Lucy EN	11	22.8.82	Died 3.11.85, age 14	Broncho-pneumonia, cardiac failure
Ada FH	15	2.12.82	Alive 1895	
Elizabeth G	5	27.10.83	Discharged 16.2.87	Improved
Florence ET	7	8.3.86	Alive 1895	
David AH	6	5.4.72	Died 1915. age 49	Late onset of blindness and deafness
Constance AW	13	31.7.86	Discharged 12.5.88	Improved
Ann MR	17	18.11.86	Discharged 26.5.91	Improved
John GT	15	6.7.74	Died 4.6.18, age 59	Alzheimer's?

were discharged with the comment 'improved', having advanced sufficiently in their social skills to be able to rejoin their families. The outcome for Down's syndrome in Langdon Down's personal series highlighted his high standard of care for his patients. When they were sick at night and he was called, he visited. When they were ill and slipping into their terminal phase, he was with them,

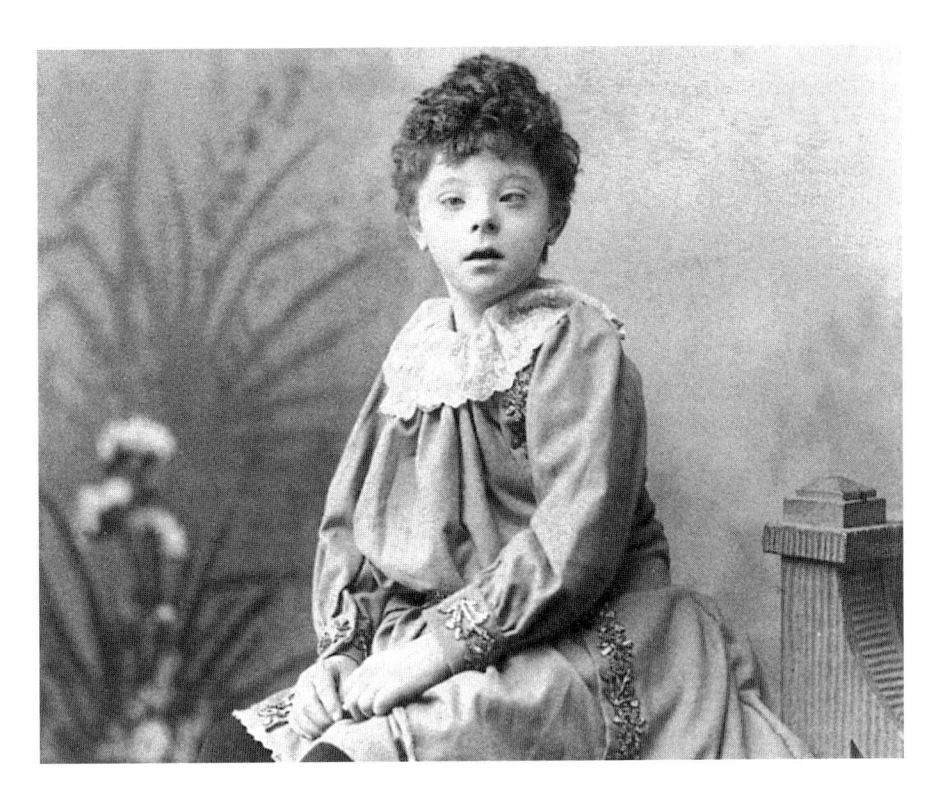

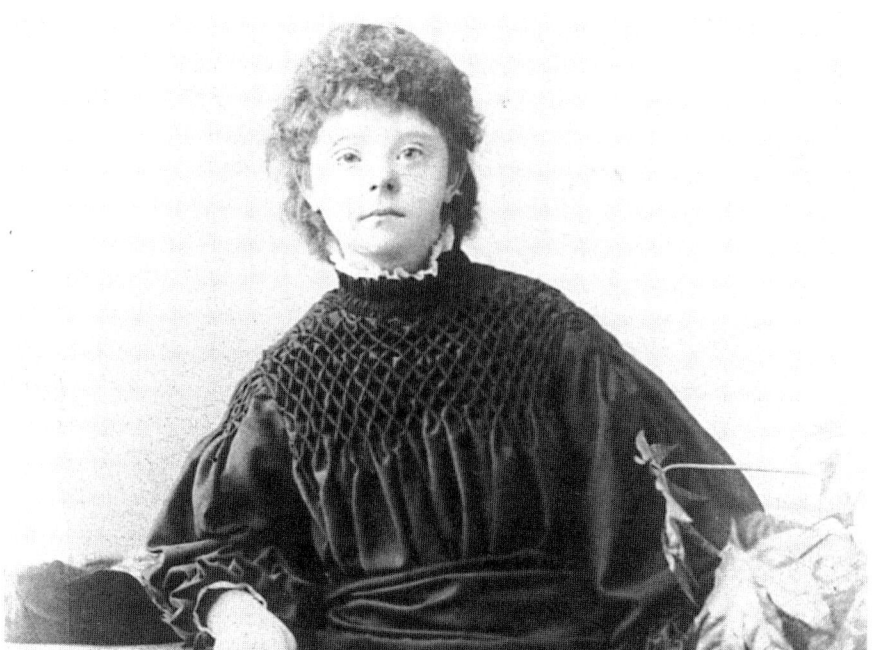

Florence T, a Down's syndrome patient at Normansfield. Photographed in 1886 when she was seven and again in 1899 aged 20.

frequently also accompanied by Mary. There is no doubt his work bore the hallmarks of the good physician.

References

1 Down JL. On idiocy and its relation to tuberculosis. *Lancet* 1867; **2**: 355–7, 391–3.
2 London Metropolitan Records Office. LMRO; H29/NF/B13/001–013. Normansfield case-books.
3 London Metropolitan Records Office. LMRO; H29/NF/B13/001.F7.

Chapter 17

The Lettsomian Lectures and Other Papers

In 1887 Langdon Down was invited by the Medical Society of London to deliver the Lettsomian Lectures. The Medical Society was a broad-based institution and prided itself on admitting physicians, surgeons and general practitioners to membership. The Lettsomian Lectures had been endowed by John Coakley Lettsom (1744–1815), a Quaker and one of the founder members of the Medical Society. He had himself written on the adverse effects of alcohol abuse and the history of medicine. The Lettsomian Lectures were the only endowed lectures organized by the Medical Society and they gave Langdon Down the opportunity of setting out his experience of almost 30 years in the field of handicap. The Lectures were widely reported in the medical press[1,2,3] and, in addition to this wide dissemination, Langdon Down published, in 1887, the three lectures together with reprints of a number of his earlier papers on disorders of the central nervous system, dating back to 1861[4].

The First Lecture

Opening the first lecture he refers to the early history of care for children who were afflicted by what he described as 'mental alienation' or 'mental incapacity'. They had been placed in the category of idiots and regarded as beyond help. He decried the Spartan-like policy of the past where there was only concern for the survival of the fittest. It had, he said, been reserved for the medicine of modern times to occupy itself with the waifs of humanity, who came under the category of the feeble in mind.

Langdon Down went on to describe how Mrs Plumbe – whose husband was later the Normansfield architect – had pressurized Dr Reed and Dr Conolly into activity in England, resulting in the setting up of homes in Highgate and Colchester and, finally, the large asylum at Earlswood. From this example other institutions had followed in England, Ireland, Scotland, the US and throughout Europe. Bearing in mind that institutions which were available did not cater for children of the poor he expressed the hope that the time was not far away when suitable provision could be made for them in the Metropolitan area.

He recognized the difficulty of cut-off points with regard to the grading of mental capacity and, in particular, the distinction between 'idiots' and 'imbeciles', terms which were in common use. He preferred the term 'feeble minded', and used the term 'imbecile' for those with dementia, comparing them to spendthrifts who had spent their fortune, in contrast to idiots who never had a fortune.

The 'Mongolian' Type

He referred again to his 1866 report, in which he identified Earlswood patients as having physical similarities to children of other races, including his description of the 'Mongolian' type – now recognized as his authoritative description of Down's syndrome – which he said had accounted for more than 10% of the feeble minded children he had seen. One new feature he mentions, not referred to in his paper on the Ethnic Classification, was the flattening at the back of the head. 'Their crania, he said, have a marked similarity. They are all brachycephalic and the posterior part is ill developed'.

He describes in detail the capacity for mimicry in children of the Mongolian type; he felt that this could be used to good effect in teaching them:

> Several patients who have been under my care have been wont to convert their pillowslips into surplices and to imitate, in tone and gesture, the clergymen or chaplain that they have recently heard. Their power if imitation is, moreover, not limited to things clerical. I have known a ventriloquist to be convulsed with laughter between the first and second parts of his entertainment on seeing a Mongolian patient mount the platform, and hearing him grotesquely imitate the performance with which the audience had been entertained. They have a strong sense of the ridiculous; this is indicated by their humorous remarks and the laughter with which they hail accidental falls, even of those to whom they are most attached. Another feature is their obstinacy – they can only be guided by consummate tact. No amount of coercion will induce them to do that which they have made up their minds not to do... Often they will talk to themselves, and they may be heard rehearsing the disputes which they think may be a feature of the following day. They are usually able to be taught to speak; speech however, is somewhat thick and indistinct and destitute of musical cadence.

There was, however, a problem with their obstinacy and he cautioned against confrontation; by avoiding orders which might provoke disobedience it was possible to maintain the appearance of authority, although it may not be possible to exercise it.

He referred to the circulation being feeble. Later writers pointed out that 50% of children with Down's syndrome had congenital heart disease, but the clinical distinction between one type of heart disease and another was only becoming apparent in the 1880s. Langdon

Down's London Hospital training had included teaching from Dr Herbert Davies, an able cardiologist of his day. However, surgical correction of cardiac defects did not become a practical proposition until the middle of the twentieth century and so the specific recognition of individual conditions was not of practical importance. The first description of the tetralogy of Fallot by his fellow member of the Pathological Society, Dr Peacock, was not published until 1870.

Langdon Down had noted that there was a family history of tuberculosis in many of the parents of Mongolian children. He took this one step further, however, and fell into the trap of ascribing the condition to the presence of a tuberculous background. He did, however, make one very important point, which was that Mongolian children did not have a long career and that very few reached adult life, being prone to succumb to serious illness or to become tuberculous like their ancestors.

Congenital Versus Acquired Disability

The importance of defining learning disability as congenital rather than acquired could cause conflict with parents. They always, he said, prefer to look for a non-congenital cause, partly because they think it important to be freed from the suspicion of hereditary influence and partly because they expect that if the condition is due to events after birth, recovery is possible. In his view learning disability provoked by accident or illness in childhood carried a worse prognosis than disability due to congenital causes. A period of 30 years experience had led him to believe that caution should be applied when giving a hopeful prognosis in children of this class. Despite their well-formed appearance and impression of normality the accidental influences were more potent for evil than many cases of malformation and deformity:

> A period of nearly 30 years has enabled me to study not only the present but the future of such children, to make a forecast based on the experience and results, and to correct the notions of sanguine hopefulness...I cannot recommend too strongly that caution should be used in giving a hopeful prognosis concerning children in this class. They may have well formed heads, finely textured skin, well chiselled mouths, sparkling eyes, features when in repose leading one to augur only brightness and intelligence. Surely, it may be thought the mind is ready to be developed from such a casket, and only time is required to ensure the thorough realisation of all ones wishes.

The Importance of Cranial Shape

In addition to the patients who showed physical abnormalities – confirming their problems as congenital – and those who had suffered from critical illnesses due to complications during birth, he classified a further group of children as having a developmental problem and describes two brothers who had lost the power of speech when they were cutting their second teeth. He had noticed in these cases that there was a very prominent ridge in the centre of the forehead and was of the opinion that this ridge was frequently associated with a tendency to neurosis. The ridge was not, he said, a cause of neurosis but its presence, like the seaweed on the seashore, was an indication of how far the tide had come over the sands. This finding would not be accepted with enthusiasm at the present time but does illustrate the thoroughness of Langdon Down's examination of his patients.

In relation to children who were found, on examination, to have a reduction in the size of their heads, he made it clear that, in his view, the smallness of the head was not due to premature fusion and early closure of the junction lines between the constituent bones of the head. He had noted, in fact, that the skull in such cases retained capacity to grow. The skull remained small only because the brain was small and the inherent defect was under-development of the brain. In this connection however he emphasized that, with regard to brain tissue, it was quality and not quantity that mattered and that the relative intelligence amongst feeble minded children could not be estimated simply by measuring the head with a tape measure and callipers. He was on the way to rejecting an association between head shape and brain function.

Polysarcia

He went on to discuss the tendency of the mentally disabled to become obese and refers to the case of polysarcia which was, in fact, the first reported case of the Prader–Willi syndrome. He described this at length in a separate paper[5] (see page 170). He had noticed that, among the learning disabled in general, the pain threshold was high and hearing and vision were frequently defective. Cataracts and colour-blindness were also sometimes seen. He also makes specific reference to a type of epilepsy characterized by salaam spasms, which one of his patients suffered from. In general he noted a delay in walking, usually until the age of three or four years and a delay in speech development.

Palate Shape

One malformation which Langdon Down thought was of special significance was the height of the arch of the palate in the mouth. This was clearly a controversial matter and not all his colleagues agreed with the emphasis which he placed on this observation. He was of the opinion that a minor defect in one generation might become more marked in the next and quoted Mr Keeling who supported this[6]. This theory was however finally rejected in 1896, the year in which he died[7]. Walter Channing came to London from Massachusetts to report on his own measurements of the palate; he had not found an abnormality in his cases; Beach had also done his own study and reached the same conclusion. Langdon Down missed this meeting of the Medicopsychological Association and died before the paper was published[8].

The Second Lecture

In this lecture Langdon Down describes the factors within pregnancy and childbirth that he had observed to affect, or cause, mental disability. He begins the discussion from a background of practical experience.

In dealing with the relative risk of instrumental delivery he noted that only 3% of his patients had been delievered using forceps but that, in up to 20% of all the idiots whose history he had investigated, there was an undoubted account of asphyxia at birth. In discussing 'suspended animation' – delayed onset of breathing leading to oxygen deprivation – he noted that delay in spontaneous breathing was frequently associated with long-term evidence of cerebral palsy. This view was based partly on his two years of hands-on experience as obstetric resident in the London Hospital. He had remained in contact with Dr Ramsbotham, the head of the obstetric department, who had confirmed that, even when forceps had been inexpertly applied, there were very few cases of cerebral lesions. Langdon Down was concerned that the use of ergot in labour might be dangerous but, with regard to labour in general, reached the important conclusion that, independently of the safety of the mother, the mental and physical ill effects to the child were more likely to be induced by prolonged pressure and delay in the use of forceps rather than by early and adroit manoeuvres.

He described various factors that seemed to have caused, or contributed to, disability in some of his patients. The first was excessively high temperatures induced by sun-stroke, which had occurred in some children passing through the Suez Canal from India. He was also suspicious of the excessive use of opium, which was frequently used in the treatment of children at that time. He mentioned the risk of child sexual abuse, which he described as erethism and which he felt both might lead to impaired psychological development but also, later, to moral delinquency.

He discounted the importance of accidental injury, but was very aware of the potential sequelae of meningitis, brain abscesses from ear infection and other disorders which might produce convulsions. He referred to many autopsies at which he had found an anaemic condition of the cerebral tissues with constriction of the blood vessels, suggesting that he had seen coning in the case of raised pressure from meningitis. The clinical condition of his own daughter Lilian who had died from prolonged convulsions must have been clear in his mind when he spoke of this subject. He mentioned, with approval, the views of Charles West of Great Ormond Street Hospital, as set out in his Lumleian Lectures, in which West had said that whatever the cause of a first fit, it could leave behind a stamp or stain which was a marker for the risk of further problems in the future.

When he goes on to discuss the causation of learning disability, he emphasizes the risk to the foetus of maternal problems in pregnancy, including uterine haemorrhage or seriously elevated temperatures. In coming to the question of inheritance he reviewed his analysis of 2000 cases. He had concluded that 84% of families had a history of neurosis of some kind and repeated his opinion that the parents of affected children frequently showed minor signs of degeneration, such as narrow palates, rabbit mouths, bad foreheads and facial exaggerations. He had looked at the question of disparity between the ages of the parents as a possible contributing factor to learning disability, but was unfortunate in his handling of statistics. He concentrated on the age disparity between the parents, but missed the opportunity of taking note of the age of the mother in his case material. So, despite having necessary data, he unfortunately failed to identify the significance of maternal age.

Returning again to the question of childbirth, he noted that 24% of those with learning disabilities and 40% of children with delayed-onset breathing, had been first-born. Having twins was not, in his experience, an important factor, but the health of the mother during pregnancy was very important. In particular he stressed the importance of emotional as well as physical health. He describes at length the importance of intemperance at the time of procreation. In this respect he was talking about the fathers' drinking habits. It did not occur to him that if the father drank heavily the mother might also and so missed the opportunity of describing the foetal alcohol syndrome. In only one of his Earlswood patients was there a clear history of maternal alcoholism but the patient concerned did not have the classical facial appearance of the foetal alcohol syndrome. In particular she lacked the totally smooth upper lip, lacking any philtrum, which is characteristic of this condition. It is, however, well-known that maternal alcoholism can affect intelligence without affecting the facial appearance.

Other Risk Factors

In attempting to explain the incidence of learning disability he described how he had studied the occupations of 400 fathers, of whom 75% were merchants, country gentlemen, army or naval officers, either of independent means or members of the aristocracy.

The remaining 25% of his patients were from families in the three learned professions – medicine, the law and the church. He made various observations in each group but they were inconclusive; his deductions were also flawed by the lack of a control group in each category.

He also devoted some discussion to the possible risk of first cousin marriages. He noted that, amongst the ancient Egyptians and Persians, incestuous marriages were common among kings and people of high rank, without any impairment or ill effect. Having extended his discussion he reached a conclusion that, if close scrutiny did not reveal any hereditary weakness, neurotic or otherwise, the facts and figures alone would not in all instances justify us in 'forbidding the banns'. Illegitimacy was rejected as a direct cause of handicap and, with regard to attempted abortion, he said that he did not have the personal experience to allow him to confirm or reject its importance.

Thyroid Deficiency

He had seen children with thyroid deficiency, some with goitre and some without. He knew their clinical appearance and identified in particular the fatty pads which developed over their collar bones, their placidity, wrinkled skin and sparse hair. He fully accepted that cretinism, with or without goitre, was due to thyroid disease and hoped that further investigation of thyroid deficiency in adults would throw light on the condition in children. The successful use of thyroid extract by mouth was not described for another 10 years and so, although he recognized the nature of cretinism, he had no treatment to offer[3].

The Role of Women in Society

He ended the lecture with some discussion about the role of women, about which he had very liberal views:

> ...there can be no reason why the faculties which they possess, should not be cultivated so as to make them not only fit to be 'mothers of men' but also companions and helpers of men. At all events let the trial be made without prejudice and let us welcome the advent of a time when women shall not be the mere frivolous toys that they are but have and enjoy the privileges and rights of which it is absurd to deprive them.

He supported the giving of the vote to women and the meetings of the 1872 National Society for Women's Suffrage were held in his Harley Street house.

Four years later, when Mrs Garrett Anderson, in the course of the campaign for the admission of women to medical school, approached the London Hospital in 1876 the reception was mixed. There was a reluctance to have men and women students in the same classes and a proposal was made to have duplicate teaching classes; when this matter came up for discussion, Langdon Down opposed the proposal. The school did have the human and material resources to run a duplicate course. His letter anticipated latter day events and the advancement of women in professions and in the Church. He may indeed have been among the first to foresee the ordination of women. His letter reads:

> Gentlemen,
>
> I have read with great care the proposals submitted by Mrs Anderson, MD, with reference to the admission of women into the wards of the London Hospital as students, and although I entertain no grave objection to women entering the Church, Law or Medicine, still I am clearly of opinion that the scheme propounded is not a practical one and that its being attempted to be carried out would prove a failure as far as the object of the applicants is concerned and would be highly detrimental, if not ruinous, to the school of the London Hospital.
>
> I am, gentlemen,
>
> >Your obedient servant,
> >
> >J Langdon Down[9].

The Third Lecture

In this lecture he talks of various specific conditions, including epilepsy, and advises methods of treatment. In addition to many general observations on learning difficulties, he also discusses his views on age-based assessment and the benefits of equal-ability education for the feeble minded. He also addresses the role of electric stimulation treatment which was then the height of fashion. Finally, he highlights one fascinating group of patients that he terms *idiots savants*.

Epilepsy

The problem of epilepsy was highlighted and he estimated that a quarter of all his patients had, at some period in their lives, been epileptic. It had been of great importance to Langdon Down to develop a good system of treatment for epilepsy at a time when there were very few options for drug therapy. Bromide and, in particular, potassium bromide had been introduced in the 1850s as the drug of choice for the treatment of epilepsy. He does not discuss treatment in his lecture but his clinical notes indicate the regime he followed, which was fairly standard at that time. If bromide failed in standard doses, the dose was raised. If this was unsuccessful additional treatment might be either with tincture of cannabis, zinc sulphate or occasionally with belladonna. It is interesting that cannabis had a recognized position as an additional therapy for epilepsy.

Physical Malformations

He had noticed that minor external congenital malformations might alert the physician to problems of handicap. In this respect he mentioned webbing of the fingers or toes, adherent ear lobules and defective formation of the ear in general. He had also noticed the tendency of the eyebrows to run over the bridge of the nose and to meet in the mid-line, a feature which is still considered to be of importance and is characteristic of the Cornelia de Lange type maldevelopment in particular. Unfortunately neither the Earlswood or Normansfield collections of photographs show any typical patients with the classical appearance of this condition.

Feeding Problems

He had also noticed how some patients were affected by rumination and that affected children brought back their food and quietly chewed it again in a bovine fashion. Pica – or the eating of rubbish, such as pebbles – was also a problem and he was aware of the possibility that a child accustomed to eating and swallowing hair could gradually accumulate a massive tangle or hair ball in the stomach, causing obstruction. Constipation likewise attracted his attention. He noted that, in the presence of tuberculosis, the cough response was reduced so the condition was less easily detected.

With regard to the identification of learning disability, he pointed out that early feeding difficulties could be a warning signal and that, later in infancy, the absence of a spontaneous muscular effort was important. Specifically he said that if there were was not a responsive leap when the feet were allowed to touch the ground, or there was no disposition to crawl, these should be noted. At a later age, the power of standing or walking might never be attained.

Age-based Assessment

He went on to make a prophetic proposal. He said that; 'in any given case we have to ask ourselves, can we in imagination put back the age two or more years and arrive thus at a time perfectly consistent with the mental condition of our patient?'[10] This suggestion he had taken from Dr Charles West, the founder of Great Ormond Street Hospital and, indeed, the testing of children by reference to an age-related standard of normality emphasized by both West and Langdon Down laid the foundations for later and more extensive and intensive system developed by Stanford and Binet. Above all else he felt that a child who did not speak by the age of six years required special consideration. He speculated that this might be due either to deafness, a local abnormality of the tongue, palate or lips, or a defect in mental power – leading to the child's inability to acquire speech because of the absence of ideas or a difficulty in converting ideas into words.

Equal-ability Education

He greatly favoured a training of children in groups of equal ability. He felt that the most successful training was affected among the child's equals; in this way healthy competition developed. He had noticed that intelligent children would not take part in the amusements or games of feeble minded ones and, in his view, the outcome of an attempt to train the feeble minded child with others more intelligent than themselves was inevitably to make their life more lonely and accentuate their condition.

He instanced a child of a nobleman who, while living in all the luxury of a well-appointed country house, was so put aside by her sisters that she never ventured on a remark and at length lost speech. He had seen the same girl, transferred to a class of children like herself, pass from monosyllabic to complete conversation. He advised against sending children with learning disability to ordinary schools, where their lives were made wretched by teasing and where they fell hopelessly behind, without the benefit of individual skill or free from the pressure of excessive competition. His concerns were to avoid having a feeble-minded child of wealthy parents dismissed to the servants quarters or, for poor parents, to avoid the dissipation of their limited energies in the management of their disabled child.

Use of Electrical Stimulation

As stated previously in his address 'The Education and Training of the Feeble in Mind', he felt that the basis of all treatment should be medical, using medical in an enlarged sense. This meant paying attention to the diet, living conditions, hygiene, muscular training, discipline and living skills. He made mention of activating feeble muscles both by massage and exercise. In his private institution in Normansfield, galvanism was certainly also tried. The famous Dr Duchenne had written a textbook on the use of electrical stimulation of the muscles by direct current[11] and this was then in fashion.

Closer to home Dr Julius Althaus had written in the *Lancet*[12] on the treatment of certain forms of paralysis with galvanic and faradic currents. He recommended that interrupted current of an alternating character was useful in treating local paralysis due to local injury of motor nerves and muscles, to reduce rheumatic effusion and in poisoning, by lead for example. He claimed that it could also have beneficial effects in paralysis from diseases of the nervous system – but only after the original lesion had subsided – and in reflex paralysis – but again only after the irritation in the spinal cord had passed.

The continuous current as delivered by galvanic batteries was, however, efficient in certain forms of paralysis due to infections of the nervous centres, particularly in those cases which had been caused by effusion in the spinal canal and incipient roughening of the cord, as well as in most instances of reflex paralysis where irritation of the cord was still present.

The apparatus for applying galvanic stimulation has survived in Normansfield, although the clinical records only refer to its use in one instance. Langdon Down however, along with many of his contemporaries, saw this form of treatment as an exciting new advance. In his address to the Royal Pharmaceutical Society, Langdon Down suggested that pharmacists might take responsibility for electrical treatments and supply them, as they did the drugs prescribed by physicians and dispensed by pharmacists. It probably had little benefit to offer but was, in his day, regarded as one of the promising modern treatments.

Idiots Savants

Langdon Down referred to the considerable number of *idiots savants* who had come under his observation. He defined them as children who, while feeble minded, exhibited special faculties which were capable of being cultivated to a great extent. In some instances the skills demonstrated could only be defined as marks of genius. He described six individuals, all male and each having a specific talent. All were probably Earlswood residents[13], as the Normansfield clinical notes do not identify any of them, although some may, of course, have been outpatients at the Royal London Hospital.

One of his *idiots savants* became so famous that he enjoyed royal patronage. He was identified by name and the details of his history and autopsy report were given in the *Journal of Mental Science* after his death[14]. This was James Henry Pullen, described as the genius of Earlswood. James Henry Pullen was born on 2 August, 1835 to parents who were first cousins. He was admitted to Essex Hall, Colchester in 1850, later moving to Earlswood[15]. His hearing was defective and he also had learning difficulties. As a child he amused himself making models of boats from chips of wood, pins and thread and, in January 1857, his Earlswood records note that he was good at drawing and that he had become a skilful carpenter.

Dr Maxwell, the Medical Superintendent entered a query: 'Is he an idiot?'. He had a good sense of numbers and, indeed, when he completed his most complex model, that of the *Great Eastern*, he made out a list of the thousands of components which he had used. Likewise he was able to keep an account of his earnings, for he was allowed to sell carvings and the administration came to query whether he was in fact doing more work for himself than for the

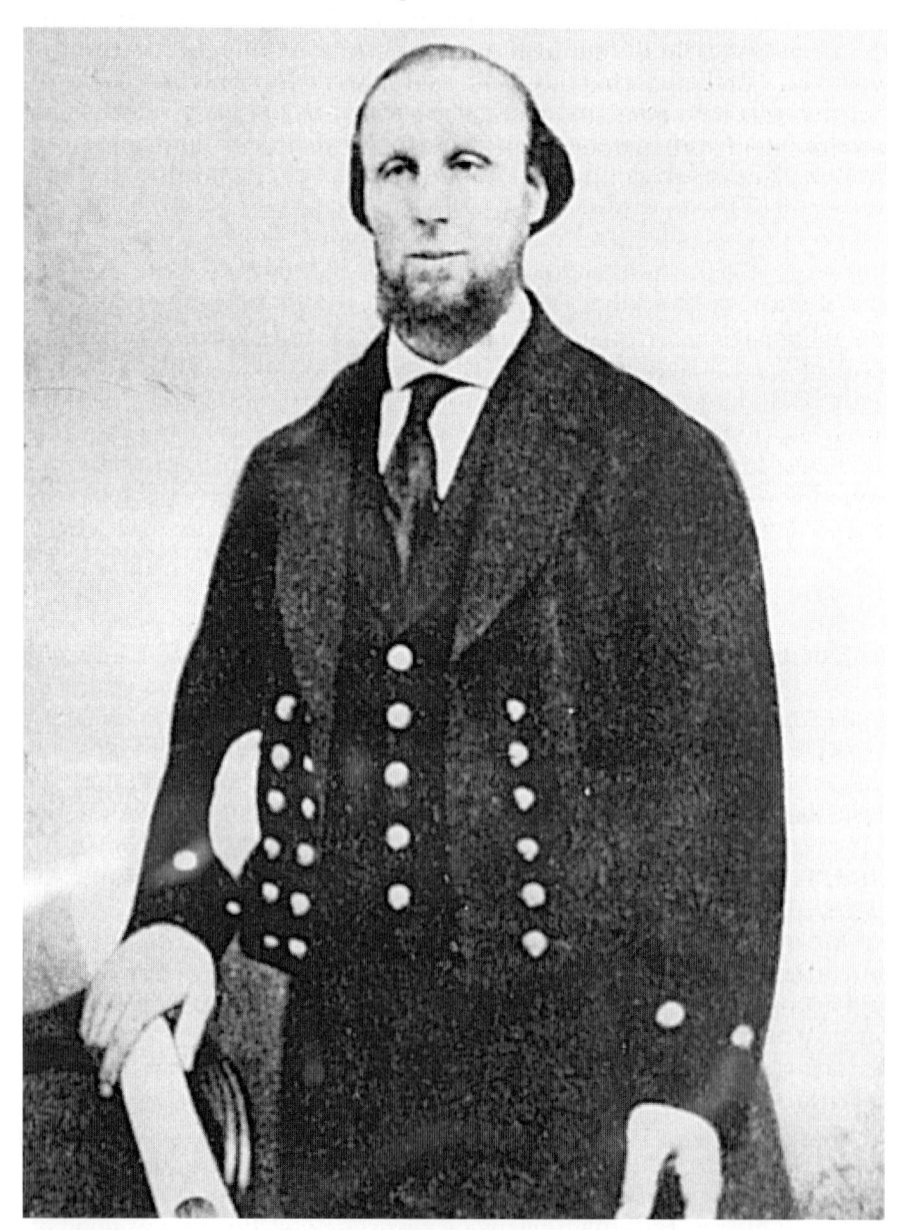

James Henry Pullen, the idiot savant *who designed the prize winning exhibit for the Paris exhibition in 1867, dressed in the admiral's uniform which he accepted in return for not pursuing his plan to marry. He also designed a realistic model of the* Great Eastern, *a famous transatlantic vessel built by Brunel.*

institution. His general understanding however would seem to have been that of a boy of about 12 years. He never learned to write sentences, but he had an extraordinary talent for numbers, in addition to his mechanical skills.

As a young man he was dissuaded from going ahead with a plan to marry a drinking companion. The Earlswood board conferred on him the fictitious title of 'admiral' and gave him a splendid uniform to wear, on condition that he remained single. His brother, William Arthur, was also admitted to Earlswood in 1862 at the age of 12. He was also deaf and, in due course, learned the deaf and dumb alphabet. William Arthur was at least as artistic as his famous brother and was eventually employed in the Earlswood printing department as a lithographic artist.

James Henry Pullen was ultimately given his own workshop. In 1881 he was employed for six months making a library cupboard for a private patient. In general he was an affable man but was subject to explosions of temper and in one of these he smashed all his handiwork and tools but also caught his leg on a rope and fractured his tibia. This was set by Langdon Down. On another occasion he developed inflammation of the left testis without any history of mumps or evidence of gonorrhoea; he may have been engaged in a brawl. He was also known to drink to excess until the last seven years of his life when the Earlswood matron persuaded him to become teetotal.

Langdon Down's most specific contact with the genius of Earlswood was in 1867. Pullen designed and constructed models of cottages which were sent to the International Exhibition in Paris. Langdon Down had hoped to attend the Exhibition but permission was refused by the Board. The Pullen exhibit was awarded a bronze medal, which was subsequently received by the Board of Management and put on display. Pullen's workmanship can still be viewed in the Royal Earlswood Museum. The most striking of his craftwork is the model of the *Great Eastern*, which took him three years to complete. The model is ten feet long, with planking fixed by almost a million and a quarter wooden pins. He had made a special pin mill to produce them. There were thirteen lifeboats on working davits and the top could be removed to show the furnishings of the state rooms. Another of his models was of an intricately rigged man-of-war. This is copper-riveted, with 42 brass cannon, two hundred pulley locks and full sail rigging. To protect his property he constructed a 13 foot high bearded monster with a mechanism for opening and shutting the mouth and eyes, striking with a sword and blowing an internal trumpet.

James Henry Pullen's autopsy report showed no identifiable ear abnormality. His brain was small, with smaller parietal, but larger temporal, lobes than a control specimen. The conclusion was that his brain was underdeveloped, with less grey matter than normal and with a simpler, less complex structure than expected. The publication of a patient's postmortem result, identifying the individual by name, was reprehensible and unethical, but this passed without comment at the time.

The second of Langdon Down's *idiots savants* who can be identified was James Thomas M[16]. He was employed to carry coals for the fire and empty slops for the kitchen maids. He had, however, an eccentric obesession with history and could, without difficulty, give a full account of the birth, life and death of any prominent person in early or ancient history. He had knowledge of all these events but did not appear to have full understanding of the occurrences he described. Dr Caldecott, then the Medical Superintendent, found that his mental powers began to decline in his sixties. In his view he suffered from high grade amentia and had the intelligence of a boy of twelve.

The question of memory intrigued Langdon Down. He referred to various individuals he had encountered – a boy who could recall the tune, the words and the number of nearly every hymn in *Hymns Ancient and Modern*, another who could name every confectioner's shop he had visited in London and the date of every visit. One knew the date of admission of every new arrival, and another the home address of every resident. Another could multiply any three figures by three with perfect accuracy, but this was his only skill; he had no memory for names and, after over two years, was still unable to remember Langdon Down's own name.

Langdon Down could make no guess about the methods by which these extraordinary skills had been developed, but did record a case of a boy whose skill in arithmetic had been lost, to some extent, following an attack of epilepsy. He had done an autopsy on one boy who had an unusual sense of time without using a clock. Langdon Down found that there was no difference between his brain and any other ordinary brain except that he had two well defined commissures or connecting tracts between the two sides of the brain. The fact that the residents with these isolated special skills did not have any unique clinical marker may have been one of the factors which led him to abandon phrenology. Most of these patients did not die during Langdon Down's lifetime and so he did not, through autopsies, become involved in the search for an associated specific structural feature of brain development, which could be said to correlate with the skills concerned.

Prader–Willi Syndrome

The Lettsomian Lectures were given in 1887 but, when they were published, Langdon Down combined with them reprints of various other papers. One of these papers[17], originally published in 1864,

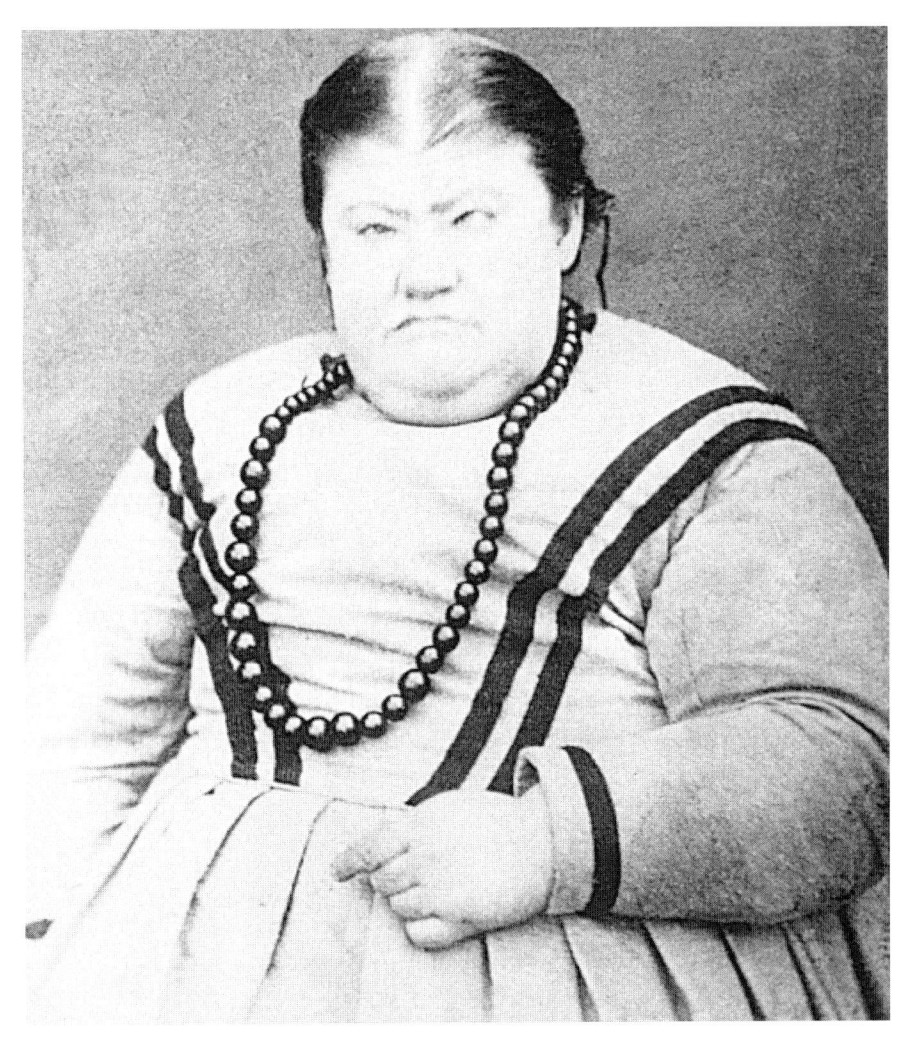

Langdon Down's patient Elizabeth C. She has the short stature, severe obesity and characteristic facial appearance of Prader–Willi syndrome.

concerned what he termed 'polysarcia', a term widely-used at the time for extreme obesity, being derived from the Greek root for excessive flesh.

One of his patients, Elizabeth C, had become grossly obese from early childhood and, at the age of 25 years, weighed 210 lbs. Her appearance was unusual, with a narrow forehead, pouting lips, downturned angles to her mouth, a squint and disproportionately small hands. She lacked muscle power and, whenever she fell, could not get up again without assistance. She had never menstruated and developed very little pubic hair. She had a voracious appetite and would lie and steal to get food. At the age of 23 she had not, as yet, learned to spell and never progressed beyond simple arithmetic but she was, however, a good needlewoman. She was only four feet, eight inches in height. She was very breathless at night and snored so deeply that the occupants of the same room were disturbed by her.

Langdon Down, having failed to reduce her weight by drug treatment, put her on a strict diet. The final drug treatment he used was Fucus Vesiculosus, specially prepared for him from dried seaweed. Conceivably the obnoxious taste of this medication might reduce the patient's appetite. He made a remarkable observation which could only have derived from his Earlswood experience. He said that the condition reminded him of that of a pig that had been spayed for fattening and concluded from this that there was ovarian insufficiency. He had no doubt seen pigs being fattened in this way when he had been in Earlswood, where there was a 150 acre farm to be supervised.

He managed to reduce her weight down with a diet which was low in fat and high in protein. She was strictly supervised and lost over four stone in weight; she maintained a steady weight of just over 10 stone until Langdon Down left Earlswood. Following Langdon Down's resignation and without his supervision and direction her weight gain accelerated once more and she died two years later. Her postmortem confirmed the forecast of ovarian insufficiency. Her ovaries were small and her uterus measured only 1.5 inches, which could be described as infantile. His forecast had been correct.

This condition and its characteristic clinical features were later described in detail in a German paper by Prader, Labhart, and Willi[18]. The disorder has since then been known as the Prader–Willi syndrome. An abnormality of chromosome number 15 is now recognized to be the cause of the condition. Accepted criteria for the diagnosis of what is currently called the Prader–Willi syndrome have been set out by a study group and reported by Dr Holm and his associates in 1990[19].

Langdon Down's patient satisfied all the major criteria of the syndrome and, in addition, suffered from the effects of the splinting of her chest movement by the overly developed fat deposits. She also had great expertise in embroidery which, in the 20th century corresponds with the unusual skill with jigsaw puzzles which has been noted in many patients. In the light of his primary observations, Langdon Down should perhaps now be recognized as the first to describe the condition[20].

In Mental Affections Langdon Down republished some 13 other papers with a neurological slant. Apart from his addresses he also published three non-neurological papers elsewhere and contributed to the understanding of the pathology of West's syndrome and Little's disease[21]. In comparative terms he was not a prolific medical writer; however Langdon Down's contribution to medical literature was nevertheless of great significance, in spite of his relatively modest output. The Lettsomian lectures have been reprinted by the McKeith Press[22] and a German translation has been published by Pies[23].

References

1. Down JL. First Lettsomian Lecture. *BMJ* 1887; **1**: 49–50.
2. Down JL. Second Lettsomian Lecture. *BMJ* 1887; **1**: 149–51.
3. Down JL. Third Lettsomian Lecture. *BMJ* 1887; **1**: 256–9.
4. Down JL. *Mental Affections of Childhood and Youth*. London: Churchill, 1887.
5. Down JL. On polysarcia and its treatment. *Lond Hosp Reports* 1864; **3**: 97.
6. Down JL. *First Lettsomian Lecture*. London: Churchill, 1887: 35.
7. Channing W. The significance of palatal deformities in idiots. *J Ment Sc* 1897; **33**: 72–86.
8. Royal London Hospital Archives.
9. Langdon Down J. *Mental Affections*. London: Churchill, 1887: 120.
10. Duchenne G-B. *De L'electrisation Localisée*. Paris: Masson, 1861.
11. Sano FF. James Henry Pullen, The Genius of Earlswood. *J Ment Sc* 1918; **64**: 251–67.
12. Althaus J. Treatment with galvanism and faradisation. *Lancet* 1865; **2**: 178–9.
13. Down JL. *Mental Affections*. London: Churchill, 1887: 99.
14. Telford Telford-Smith. Cases of sporadic cretinism treated by thyroid extract. *J Ment Sc* 1895; **30**: 280–89.
15. Surrey Record Office. SRO. Patient casebooks 392/1/2/2
16. Down JL. *Mental Affections*. London: Churchill, 1887: 167–80.
17. Prader A, Labhart A, Willi H. Ein Syndrom Van Adipositas etc. *Schweiz Med Wochenschr* 1956; 867; 1260–1.
18. Prader–Willi Syndrome: Consensus Diagnostic Criteria. *Pediatrics* 1990; **91**: 398–400.
19. Down JL. *On Some Mental Affections of Childhood and Youth, being the Lettsomian Lectures Delivered Before the Medical Society of London in 1887, together with Some Other Papers*. London: Blackwell Science, 1990.
20. Ward OC. Langdon Down's 1864 case of Prader–Willi syndrome. *J Roy Soc Med* 1997; 90: 694–6.
21. Ward OC. John Langdon Down (1828–1896). In: Rose C, ed. *A Short History of Neurology*. London: Butterworth. In press.
22. Down JL. Mental Affections of Childhood and Youth. In: Mitchell R, ed. *Classics in Developmental Medicine, No. 5*. McKeith Press, 1990.
23. Pies NJ. *Ein Pionier der Sozielpadiatrie. John Langdon Haydon Langdon Down (1828–1891)*. Karlsruhe: G Braum, 1996.

Chapter 18

Down's Influences and Beliefs

John Langdon Down was a simple man. He had read no textbooks on philosophy and his prize essay in Torpoint on 'The Benevolence of the Almighty[1]' portrays him as someone who believed in the reality of an Almighty God, who had created mankind with the distinguishing attribute of a spirit or soul. Against a background of these traditional beliefs he was also, however, a man of his time.

Religion and Darwinism

The evolution process proposed by Darwin was the backdrop against which all scientific discussions took place. According to the thinking of his age the races of mankind, identifiable by different physical characteristics, represented stages in evolution, with the most sophisticated culmination represented in the Caucasian white races. Down's view was that the racial boundaries were not irrevocably fixed. Charles Darwin believed that natural selection may demand a hard human struggle for survival but also that the laws of morality demanded aid and compassion for the weak and helpless. He said 'We cannot check our sympathy even at the urging of hard reason, without deterioration in the noblest parts of our nature... if we were intentionally to neglect the weak and helpless, it could only be for a contingent benefit, with an overwhelming present evil'[2]. Darwin accepted however that, as in the animal world, there was a hierarchy of cultural perfection in man:

> Man, like every other animal, has no doubt advanced to its present high condition through a struggle for existence consequent on his rapid multiplication; and if he is to advance higher still, it is to be feared that he must remain subject to a severer struggle. Otherwise we would sink into indolence and the more gifted men would not be successful in the battle for life than the less gifted[3].

In 1872 in his *The Expression of the Emotions*[4] he did, however, set out to show that all the chief gestures and expressions of emotion exhibited by man are the same throughout the world, which afforded a new argument in favour of the several races of man being descended from a single parent stock and further, that these expressions resembled in many important particulars the movements and gestures of animals[4]. Despite this, it was widely held that Caucasian races represented the acme of developmental perfection, although Darwin himself did not say this.

Herbert Odom in his 'Generalisations on Race in Nineteenth Century Physical Anthropology' emphasized the importance of the concept of race in the 1850s and quotes Benjamin Disraeli as saying; 'Race implies difference, difference implies superiority, and superiority leads to predominance'[5]. This concept had been the breaking point in the London scientific world at the time. The Anthropological Society saw the human races as being fixed and immobile and, on this account, asserted that slaves in the US, if freed, would stay and may even enjoy continuing to be slaves[6]. Langdon Down was opposed to the concept of slavery and criticized the American anthropologists Nott and Gliddon who, as he said; 'laboured to prove that the various ethnic families were distinct species, and a strong argument was based on this to justify a certain domestic institution'[7]; the institution was slavery. The diversion of the offspring of one ethnic group into another group with different ethnic characteristics meant that the ethnic groups were of the same stock.

For Langdon Down however, as for many of his contemporaries, there was an impossible chasm between the ape or the chimpanzee and mankind. Addressing the British Medical Association in 1887, Langdon Down said that, having found representatives of different racial appearance among his disabled patients, showing as it did the possibility of degeneration from higher to lower levels of development, he was convinced of man's descent from a single couple, as described in Genesis[8].

A great debate ranged among those who felt that Darwinism ran counter to the specific description of the creation of the world, its creatures and man in the Genesis description in the Old Testament but, for Langdon Down, there was no argument. There was a further debate which had its origin in the views of Richard Whateley, Archbishop of Dublin, who felt that the lesser or inferior races were fixed in a time warp in which they could neither advance nor improve under their own momentum[9]. Langdon Down did not accept this position and believed there was always room for improvement by stepwise training.

In this he followed Thelwall who wrote, in 1810, that he perceived the problem in learning disability to be one of a lack of stimulatory input into the mind, which remained 'contracted in its sphere of activity by physical privation'[10]. Thelwall believed that this lack could be overcome by an increased sensory input. Langdon Down shared this view[11]. Langdon Down's positive view was repeated by others such as Bucknill, who took an optimistic view that the helpless imbecile could 'be educated up to the point which renders it possible to introduce him to the social life of our time as an independent and efficient man'[12]. He was more optimistic than many of the traditional experts, Esquirol for instance believing that the lowest level of intellect was incapable of improvement[13].

Religious Implications of Disability

One of the influences on Langdon Down was the French physician Benedict Morel (1809–73). Morel had written extensively on moral treatment; by this he meant giving moral support, supplemented by using the strong will of a therapist to ensure compliance of the trainee in all matters of re-education. He regarded downgrading of man's stature as a by-product of the fall from grace of the human race. Adam and Eve had been responsible for the first fall from the state of perfection after they had disobeyed a single prohibition and degenerated from perfection. This perception of a biological flaw took up an older concept that a handicapped person was, to a degree, considered a changeling or incomplete person. This was an even more fundamental aberration than that of Knox. He claimed that the various races known throughout recorded history were, effectively, distinct species and that they must be ranged on a scale according to their civilizational aptitudes. This at least allowed of a child with Down's syndrome being assigned a position in the human hierarchy, albeit on a lower rung of the ladder[14].

The distinction between insanity and learning disability was still blurred and, although Langdon Down was one of those who was at the forefront in advocating that the two should be separated, he nevertheless still adhered to the older view that, at least in relation to causation, the two were connected. He ended his third Lettsomian Lecture with a tribute to, amongst others, Samuel Howe. Howe had reported to the Legislation of Massachussets on Idiocy in 1848 and was of the opinion that the causes of idiocy were multiple but that; 'among the progenitors of the sufferers there is found a degree of physical degeneration, and a mental and moral darkness, which will scarce to be credited'[15] Langdon Down had read Howe's report and was influenced by his analysis of the causation of handicap.

Howe also wrote a supplement to the report, in which he said:

The moral to be drawn from the existence of the individual idiot is this – he, or his parents, have so far violated the natural laws, so far marred the beautiful organism of the body, that it is an unfit instrument for the manifestations of the powers of the soul ... they disregard the conditions which should be observed in inter-marriage; they overlook the hereditary transmission of certain morbid tendencies, and they pervert the natural appetites of the body into lusts of diverse kinds, the natural motions of the mind in to fearful passions, and thus bring down the awful consequences of their own ignorance and sin upon the heads of their unoffending children[15].

The Langdon Downs read a great deal about religion and religious history and ultimately moved from their starker Nonconformist affiliation towards the Church of England.

Racial Implications of Disability

John Langdon Down could not live when he lived and remain untouched by the ideas of the time. He was ambivalent about Darwinism and its implied fixed gradation of the human races; he understood it, but did not like the fact that it was being used by some to justify racial discrimination. In his direct reference to religion he used a delicate touch and clearly did not wish to impose his views on others. His own view of the human race was that it was all one, as he had stated in his Ethnic Classification[16] although, in his labelling of all the different ethnic types he lost sight of what he had originally observed – that the largest number of children with congenital learning disability were of the Caucasian type. His great interest in the patients with identifiable and distinguishing physical characteristics led him away from the necessity to explain the large Caucasian group who had no stigmata.

Langdon Down had had some contact with theologians. This is to be expected as his eldest sister, Jane, had married one of the most distinguished Congregational preachers of her day, the Reverend David Everard Ford. In his first Lettsomian Lecture he refers with approval to Charles West's suggestion that prior illness could leave behind a mark or stamp 'not unlike what theologians tell as of the flaw which our first parents sin has left upon her moral nature – a pre-disposition in short to a great evil'[17]. The degeneracy was frequently a gradual process, affecting individuals with increasing intensity through a number of generations. This concept of gradual degeneration was one that was widely accepted in his own time; he referred to in his first Lettsomian Lecture when he spoke of the appearance of increasing deformity of the palate observed in a family over three generations. Finding insanity or purported insanity in the family tree was taken, like a history of tuberculosis, as being evidence of degeneracy.

Langdon Down was a practical idealist prepared to live out the principles in which he believed, combining scientific observation with concern for his patients, their families and future. For him his Ethnic Classification was a clinical tool. He followed the concepts of Robert Dunn, who at a meeting of the Ethnological Society on 3rd February, 1863 said:

> A genus Homo was one... on the ground that in man's moral and religious attributes the inferior animals do not participate; it was this, he considered, that constitutes the difference between him and them. The barrier was thus... impassable between man and

the chimpanzee and gorilla; and forever two handed and two footed man, in his erect attitude and with his articulate voice is found his claims to a common humanity must be immediately acknowledged, however debased the type may be or mean the garb in which humanity is closed[18].

It was Dunn's conviction 'that there was proof of a general unity exhibited in all the races of the great family of man; in so much as they were all endowed with the same instinctive, sensational, perceptive and intellectual faculties – the same mental activities however much they vary in degree'[18].

Dunn believed however that the learning processes were different in the various races and thought that Negro children could not successfully be educated with white children for this reason. Langdon Down perceived that because he had seen children with Down's syndrome excel in mimicry this special attribute could be used to advance their education generally. For Langdon Down the identification of the Mongolian child was important because 'the improvement which training effects in them is greatly in excess of what would be predicted if one did not know the type'[19]. The races of mankind were different and the children of different races might benefit from different approaches to training.

Nowhere did Langdon Down ever concede that learning disability was the result of regression to a sub-human level. Unfortunately his son, Reginald, thought otherwise; he started a thesis which, had it been accepted, would have dismissed the individuals with Down's syndrome as lesser beings (see Chapter 15). The closest Langdon Down came to this was in his third Lettsomian lecture when he described the brain of a microcephalic child as showing, in part, the simplicity of a 'quadrumanous' type, ie resembling that of a four-footed animal, but concluded that the overall features of the brain were essentially human. In the end he abandoned his ethnic concept, but he had sown the seed that was to become a basis for the division of children with learning disability into different scientific categories.

Conolly, Séguin and Blumenbach

John Conolly is best remembered for his humanitarian efforts on the part of the insane. He also made a great impact on Langdon Down. He had been London University's first Professor of Medicine prior to taking up an appointment as Medical Superintendent of the Middlesex County Pauper Lunatic Asylum at Hanwell in 1839. Here he immediately abolished all forms of personal restraint, going on to change the whole character of the asylum, introducing a regime of regular exercise, rest, diversionary occupations and the psychological control of aberration. His ambition was to abolish all restraint so that the 'lunatic' could gain the dignity of a sick human being; he said that when a patient was tied up, all regard for him ceased. His aim was 'to control the violent without anger, soothe the irritable without weak and foolish concessions, cheer and comfort the depressed, guard the imbecile and impulsive and direct all'[20].

When his health failed he left Hanwell and, from the following year, he was closely associated with the Reverend Andrew Reed in the development of an institution for the learning disabled. Their motivation was Christian and they aimed to follow St Paul's instruction: 'Now I exhort you brethren, warn them that are unruly, comfort the feeble minded, be patient to all men'[21].

Conolly had visited Paris in 1845 and there met the famous Edouard Séguin. When Séguin went to the US in 1850 he remained in contact and visited Earlswood in 1856, accompanied by Dr Howe of Boston. Séguin was a great reformer and had developed what he described as the moral treatment for the learning disabled. Kraft has reviewed this at length[22]. The moral treatment was essentially based on non-restraint and the development of basic exercises to do with motor control. The pupil was to imitate the teacher in various drills. The sense of touch was to be intensively developed. Séguin hoped that the observation of the learning disabled 'from the cradle to the slab'[23] would throw new light on the study of anthropology, a concept to which Conolly also subscribed. The moral treatment was overdue. There was at the time an overall public attitude of disgust, apathy, indifference and shame leading to the persecution of the mentally ill. Kraft describes them as being whirled in gyrators, drenched under cold showers, copiously bled, manacled, leeched and drastically purged. Heavy use was made of emetics and narcotics and there was brutal confinement and massive restraint[24]. The description of the new regime as the 'moral treatment' was intended to contrast with the physical treatment; in its presentation it reflected humanitarianism, occupational therapy, non-restraint and what might be described as tender loving care.

Conolly had never worked directly with the learning disabled but was a Visitor to the Royal Earlswood Asylum for Idiots – the successor to Park House, the first of Andrew Reed's asylums. Langdon Down contributed to Dr James Clark's Memoir of John Conolly. In this he said of Conolly:

> His visits were the most refreshing incidents of my recollection in connection with the asylum. Entering on my work as an untried man, and finding myself allied to an institution which had become unpopular at the Lunacy Board, I was mainly decided on holding a position which had so much to overwhelm me by the influence of Dr Conolly. That influence was magical. The humility of his character was only equalled by the real love he manifested for the mentally afflicted... For myself, I have often

had to seek his counsel, and never without being struck by his judgement and the fascination of his influence, the high resolve he inspired in one and what willingness he exhibited to maintain coequally with the responsibility, the power of the medical superintendent and thus prevent a repetition of those evils which he had so bitterly to lament in his own experience[23].

Conolly was an eloquent speaker and Clark includes in his memoir a part of Conolly's speech to a public meeting in Cambridge in support of the Royal Earlswood Asylum. In the course of it he said of his visits to the homes of candidates for admission to the asylum:

After some search the family is found in some obscure and unhealthy locality, where from wanton ignorance every neglect exists which invites every physical and moral evil; everything that seems to solicit epidemic diseases to settle and spread there, and to ask the cholera to come and all the scrofulous forms of deterioration to abide, and all the disfigurements of the human form and human mind to manifest themselves. In damp rooms, in close and noisome courts or in desolate unventilated apartments, reached by no inviting stair, are to be found residing, forever toiling, the parents who have applied for assistance.

Parents who have shown this anxiety are usually industrious, but very poor. The father works at some handicraft business, and his wife is engaged in washing, or in some ill-liberally remunerated work, as shoe binding or waistcoat making, or perhaps shirt making. They must work or starve. The know no holidays; for if they cease to work they and their little children must cease to eat, cease to have a fire to warm them, clothes to cover them or any kind of bed to sleep upon. The house seems generally very full of children, not yet old enough to work and who are yet unconscious that their lot in life is mere labour; and whose appearance is often so delicate and attractive as to form a strange contrast with the things around them[24].

He goes on to discuss the lot of an imbecile child:

...the poor imbecile remains alone, and becomes an even heavier burden to its father and mother when years are gathering over them. With all that they can do the child grows only a stronger animal; learns to walk about, but is uninstructed, uncontrolled, helpless; if possessed of much energy the dread of its neighbours; and if quiet and timid, hunted from street to street and exposed to every kind of wanton cruelty[24].

Conolly became a great enthusiast for Séguin's method of education by kindness; discipline was enforced only by the threat of deprivation of approval. When Langdon Down was appointed to Earlswood as the Medical Superintendent it was Conolly who developed his enthusiasm for Séguin's methods. It was very unfortunate that, in 1864, when Séguin requested a period of sabbatical accommodation with Langdon Down, the Board of Earlswood refused him.

Conolly's impact on John Langdon Down furthered two specific projects. Séguin had suggested that anthropological research might be based on the study of groups of mentally disabled children. Langdon Down began to study the configuration of the head. He used a textbook written by Combe and cut out the numerical table for reference[25]. Conolly had already put in place a system for the measurement of the various dimensions of the head in the patients in Park House, the forerunner of Earlswood. The system was carried on in Earlswood and, when Langdon Down took up his appointment, head measurements were already standard. This indeed led to his identification of the flattening of the back of the head in Down's syndrome.

The second major influence that Conolly had on Langdon Down was the introduction of photography. Conolly had written a series of papers on the 'Physiognomy of insanity' in the *Medical Times and Gazette* in 1858–9 based mainly on lithographs of clinical photographs taken by Dr Hugh Welch Diamond[26]. Diamond was, indeed, a member of the Medico-Psychological Association from as early as 1851. He never presented his work at the Medico-Psychological Association formally, but Langdon Down and he clearly knew each other and he appears on a guest list at Langdon Down's home in Normansfield in 1870. Conolly, having worked with Diamond on the use of photography, came to follow the same interest with Langdon Down.

Langdon Down also came to share Conolly's interest in anthropology. Working together they set about endeavouring to look for anthropological traits in the Earlswood residents, walking the wards together and trying to identify residents with specific racial characteristics. Langdon Down developed these ideas and the result was the 'Ethnic Classification' which he published in 1866. Conolly and he were kindred spirits, working together in close harmony, sharing the same religious conviction, expectation and optimism, matched by enthusiasm for new developments.

Even before he had entered the psychiatric service, Conolly had developed an enthusiasm for ethnology; a branch of anthropology that sought to find a correlation between the faculties of man and specific local anatomical areas in the brain. Recognizing the possibility that different configurations of the skull might be an indication of the relative development of the assumed brain centres for different faculties led to a search for identifying features which could point to strengths or weaknesses in character. Phrenology swept through the scientific community in

Great Britain in the early Victorian years[27]. There were many papers written on the subject and it was conceived that the different contour lines of different races might indicate differences in their psychological make-up[28]. Phrenology came under attack from religious authorities, mainly on the basis that it implied that man was self-contained and this his reactions were predetermined by the degree of development of different cerebral functions. Additionally, religious authorities objected to the implication that the immortal soul could be identified and located in a specific area of the brain. It was scientific evidence however which led to its eventual rejection; Roget, in the *Encyclopaedia Britannica*, stated that localization of brain function had never been confirmed and that, additionally, there was no necessary connection between the external configuration of areas of the brain and the overlying skull surface[29]. The philosophy of phrenology was dismissed as speculative.

In 1865, the year in which he carried out his photographic review, the Anthropological Society of London reprinted the papers of Friedrich Blumenbach. The Bendyshe translation included a selection from Blumenbach's engravings of a typical selection of skulls of various races, which he described as Caucasian, Mongolian, Ethiopic, American and Malay. Blumenbach had written a vigorous rebuttal of the concept that the Negro race was inferior, quoting Fuller – a highly educated Negro – who had said that the Negro was in 'God's image, although made out of ebony'. Blumenbach dismissed the concept that racial skeletal differences could be equated with any downgrading of intelligence. He spoke of the good disposition and faculties of the black brethren, their tenderness of heart and the examples of great intellectual accomplishments among their race[30].

The Bendyshe translation was on Langdon Down's 1865 personal booklist. It may have been his recognition that acceptance of the principles of ethnology could imply the acceptance of slavery which led Langdon Down to publicly abandon his support for ethnology. Zihni, reviewing Langdon Down's impact, has reached the same conclusion[31]. Langdon Down refers specifically to the question of slavery in his first Lettsomian lecture. His original interest in ethnology had, however, led to his ethnic review of the Earlswood patients and from there to the specific identification of Down's syndrome. This was to be all that remained of his dalliance with ethnology, apart from his photographs and collection of cranial specimens collected at autopsy. When he established his own centre in Normansfield, he abandoned head measurements. In practice he had found skull measurements to be unreliable but, in the first instance, the measurements had contributed to the recognition of Down's syndrome. Conolly died in 1866 and never had to face his protegé's rejection of his ideas.

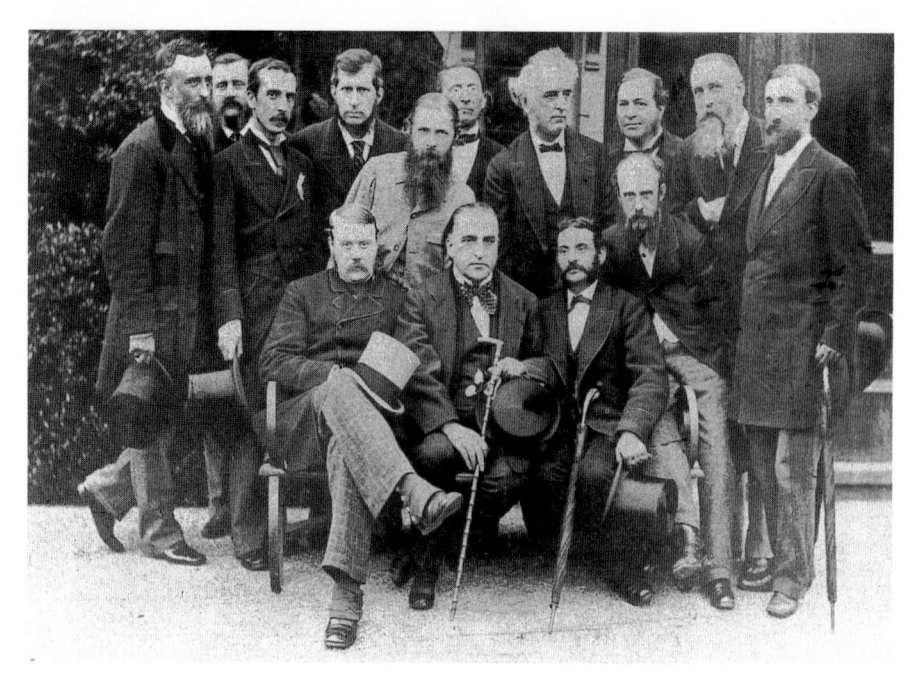

Langdon Down with members of the British Medical Association in 1895, when he entertained 500 guests at Normansfield. He was founder President of the South Thames Branch.

Learned Societies

John Langdon Down was a member of a very large number of learned societies. These included the Anthropological, Medico-Psychological, Neurological, Pathological, and New Sydenham Societies. On the wider stage, he was the Founder President of the Thames Valley Branch of the British Medical Association. In all of these he was a liberal-minded, reliable insider.

In the Medical Society of London he was a regular attender. He was Vice President in 1885 and 1886, a member of Council in 1887 and on the Committee of Referees in 1888. He went to Belfast for the meeting of the British Medical Association in 1884 and it is recorded that he spoke at the section of psychology on the management of the idiot and imbecile child. There is, however, no published report of this either in the Belfast newspapers or the contemporary medical journals. Mounting pressures on his time began to intrude on his academic activities. The tragic death of his son Everleigh also affected him. From the 1880s onwards he published no new papers and his attendance at the learned societies with which he was associated were relatively low profile.

References

1   Down JL. *Nature's Balance*. Crockford's, 1852.

2 Darwin C. *Life and Letters*, Vol 2. London: John Murray, 1888: 383.
3 Darwin C. *Descent of Man*. London: John Murray, 1888: 618.
4 Obituary, *Lancet* 1882; **1**: 712–14.
5 Odom HH. Generalisations on race. *Isis* 1967; **58**: 5–18.
6 Editorial. *BMJ* 1865; **1**: 462.
7 Down JL. *Mental Affections*. London: Churchill, 1887: 8.
8 *Surrey Comet*. 9 July 1887.
9 Gelb SA. The Beast in Man: Degenerationism and Mental Retardation 1900–1920. *Mental Retardation* 1995; **33**: 1–9.
10 Thelwall J: *Imperfect Development of the Faculties, Mental and Moral*. London: Richard Taylor, 1810.
11 Down JL. *The Education and Training of the Feeble in Mind*. London: Lewis, 1876: 14.
12 Bucknill JC. Address on Idiocy. *J Ment Sc* 1873; **29**: 169–83.
13 Esquirol JED. *Mental Maladies*. Philadelphia: Lea and Blanchard, 1845.
14 Morel B. *Traité des Dégénérescences Physiques Intellectuelles et Morales de L'espèce Humaines*. Paris: Baillière, 1857.
15 Howe SG. *Report to the Legislature of Massachusetts upon Idiocy*. Boston: Coolidge and Wiley, 1848.
16 Down JL. Observations on an Ethnic Classification of Idiots. *London Hospital Reports*. 1862; **3**: 259–62.
17 Down JL. *Mental Affections*. London: Churchill, 1887: 28.
18 Dunn R. On the psychological differences which exist among the typical races of man. *BMJ* 1863; 1: 175–7.
19 Down JL. Third Lettsomian Lecture. *BMJ* 1887; **1**: 256–9.
20 Hunter R. One hundred years after John Conolly. *Proc Roy Soc of Med* 1967; **60**: 85-9.
21 The Bible. New Testament. St Paul's letter to the Thessalonians. 1; **5**: 14.
22 Kraft I. Edouard Séguin and the 19th century Moral Treatment of Idiots. *Bull Hist Med* 1961; **35**: 393–418.
23 Clark J. *A Memoir of John Connolly*. London: John Murray, 1860.
24 Clark J. *A Memoir of John Conolly, MD, DCL*. London: John Murray, 1869.
25 Combe G. *Outline of Phrenology*. 7th Edition. Edinburgh: McLaughlan and Stewart, 1859.
26 Conolly J. The Physiognomy of Insanity, *Med Times Gaz*. 1858–9; **16**: 2–4, et seq.
27 Parsinnen TM. Popular Science & Society; The phrenology movement in early Victorian Britain. *J Soc Hist* 1974; **8**: 1–20.
28 Minchin H. Contributions to craniology. *Quart J Med Sc* 1856: 1–26.
29 Roget PM. Treatises of Physiology and Phrenology. *Encyclopaedia Britannica 1838*. Edinburgh: Black.

30 Bendyshe T. *The Anthropological Treatises of Johann Friedrich Blumenbach*. London: Longman Green, 1865.
31 Zihni L. *Unpublished D. Phil thesis: History of the Relationship between the Concept and Treatment of People with Down's Syndrome in Britain and America 1866–1967*. University College London, 1990.

Chapter 19

The Langdon Down Photographs

John Langdon Down was an innovative man. He was among the first to consider the installation of electricity and, when he bought the lease of 81 Harley Street, this was one of the first things he did. He had a good knowledge of physics and electricity and, from an early stage, photography appealed to him. He bought his own camera and took his first clinical photograph in 1862; this was a difficult process at the time as photography had only become an established procedure around 1845.

When he came to leave the Royal Earlswood Hospital for Idiots the management had endeavoured to establish a procedure for the records that included the use of photographs; this was due directly to Langdon Down, who had instituted this practice during his time there. We do not know precisely what camera John Langdon Down used. What is certain is that he showed remarkable control and exhibition of persuasive powers in encouraging his restless subjects to remain still for long enough to allow for exposures which, unlike today, were of very long duration. He was clearly happy with his camera's performance for he does not appear to have changed it for over 15 years.

Cameras at that time were little more than well-constructed, light-proof wooden boxes with provision at one end for glass plates and at the other for lenses, in sliding, geared tubes to allow for focusing. He used what was described as the wet collodion process. Frederick Scott Archer, who had devised the process, introduced a camera specifically designed to simplify the long and tedious process involved and this is what Langdon Down may have used. Langdon Down had his own dark-room in Normansfield, partitioned off from the pharmacy building.

Glass plates were not commercially available and, initially, John Langdon Down would have had to cut them to size himself, possibly using the hospital workshop. Then, immediately before a photographic session, a sticky solution of iodized collodion sensitized with silver nitrate had to be run as evenly as possible over the individual plates. The plates were exposed in the camera while still 'tacky'. They were then removed and developed in pyrogallic and acetic acid solution, fixed in hypochlorite or potassium cyanide and finally washed and dried. The alternative to the collodion process was the calotype method but, as this required even longer exposures, he is unlikely to have used it.

Exposing the negative was only the first stage. He may have developed the negatives by coating plain paper with egg white and salt, sensitized it with silver nitrate and then printed by exposure in daylight to the negative in a two-part hinged frame. The print could be viewed to assess its stage of development and after this it would be fixed, washed and dried. All the negatives show a defect in the left upper corner, where there is a small circular imprint. This is where Langdon Down held a glass plate between his forefinger and his thumb while he applied the chemical solution.

At the time he began his photographic survey there were 428 residents in the Royal Earlswood Hospital. In 1862 he took 44 photographs, the names of 34 of his subjects being hatched in the right hand corner of the negative glass plate. None of these patients were photographed subsequently when he extended the series in 1865. The 1862 series included two photographs of his son Everleigh aged four months, another of Everleigh with his mother and another photograph which is probably that of Mrs Sarah Crellin, Langdon Down's sister, who played such an important role in the early days of his career. The death of Lilian and a preoccupation with an outbreak of measles brought the study to a halt for the time being. There are, partly as a result of this, no surviving photos of either Reginald or Percival as babies or children.

In 1865 he progressed to using larger plates; the negatives of 206 photographs survive. In 1912 his son, Reginald, who was also interested in photography, conducted a photographic survey of the Normansfield residents. He also appears to have reviewed his father's collection of photographs a few years later, as they were stored interleaved with newspaper dated 1916; he may perhaps have wished to compare his father's work with his own. By this time photography had become an art as well as a craft; it was now an industry. Prepared glass plates, factory coated and using an emulsion similar to that in use today were readily available; roll-film was also being used, though mainly by amateurs. This was the result of the Eastman Kodak Company's work and their awareness of the huge potential in cameras for the novice photographer.

Langdon Down's glass negatives were subsequently dispersed. Lord Christopher Brain, John Langdon Down's great-grandson, passed 154 of these to the archives department of the Great Ormond Street Hospital for review in 1984, where the negatives were cleaned, packaged and catalogued by the archivist Ray Lunnon. The balance of the negatives remained in a basement room in Normansfield Hospital. It was an exciting occasion when, during a preliminary biographic survey of Normansfield in 1995, the cardboard boxes containing the balance of the Earlswood photographs were located. There were 52 of these in total and, fortunately, no duplication between the Great Ormond Street collection and the new Normansfield discovery. The two series have now been integrated for analysis by Ken Simmons, archival photographer at the Surrey Records Office.

Langdon Down never went on to produce slides for projection from his photographic series and, although Normansfield acquired a magic lantern in 1873, projection for clinical purposes does not appear to have been developed. This was possibly due to the greater complexity of the photographic procedure involved in making slides. Magic lantern shows were in fact held for the residents and staff but, whenever visiting medical groups came to Normansfield, they met with individual residents rather than being shown their photographs.

Langdon Down spoke of his 'Mongolian' group as representing 10% of his case load, but unfortunately only about 10 photos still remain that probably show patients affected by Down's syndrome. It may be that others were lost or misplaced over the years. The photographs in general are those of cheerful, relaxed and friendly subjects, very few of them showing signs of reluctance or disinterest.

Langdon Down produced an experimental series of prints, which he made and processed himself. There are 36 relating to the 52 Normansfield negatives and 91 relating to the Great Ormond Street collection of 154 negatives. He retained the negatives and subsequently had commercial prints made of about half of these. Searching through the series for specific points of interest, one patient does indeed show signs of facial paralysis. (No. 141). Another is clearly microcephalic, (no name, no number), with a very small head size and the presence of a number with clinical features of Down's syndrome has been mentioned.

As a historical archive the collection is of great importance. It is also of importance in relation to the manner in which Langdon Down reached his conclusions about the similarity of facial structures in individual groups. The difficulty in identifying all the sub-groups which he mentioned, Mongolian, Ethiopian and Malaysian, may relate to the fact that the best examples of these were retained in some other collection, which, like his notebooks, have not survived. There is a consecutive gap in the series from 239–72. These may be the missing ethnic types. He may, however, have been carried away by enthusiasm for the project and so over-emphasized minor facial variations which, to another observer, are less convincing.

Langdon Down deserves great credit for the dedication and persistence which resulted in the assembly of such a large and representative body of clinical material. The question might by asked why he did not continue to complete his review of the Earlswood residents; he stopped after photographing just over half the patients. It may be that he realized that he had already accumulated such a large body of material that it would be difficult for him to process and analyse it. Alternatively, growing pressures of clinical responsibility at the time of Earlswood's expansion may have made it impossible for him to proceed single-handed with further investigation. The death of Lilian may also have slowed him down. The records indicate that he had no help, except for possibly Mr Sanders, the Assistant Medical Officer, although he may also have been helped by Mary.

He certainly received no financial assistance from the Board and, under the circumstances, his photographic collection was indisputably his personal as well as his intellectual property. When he left Earlswood he took the collection with him. One of the

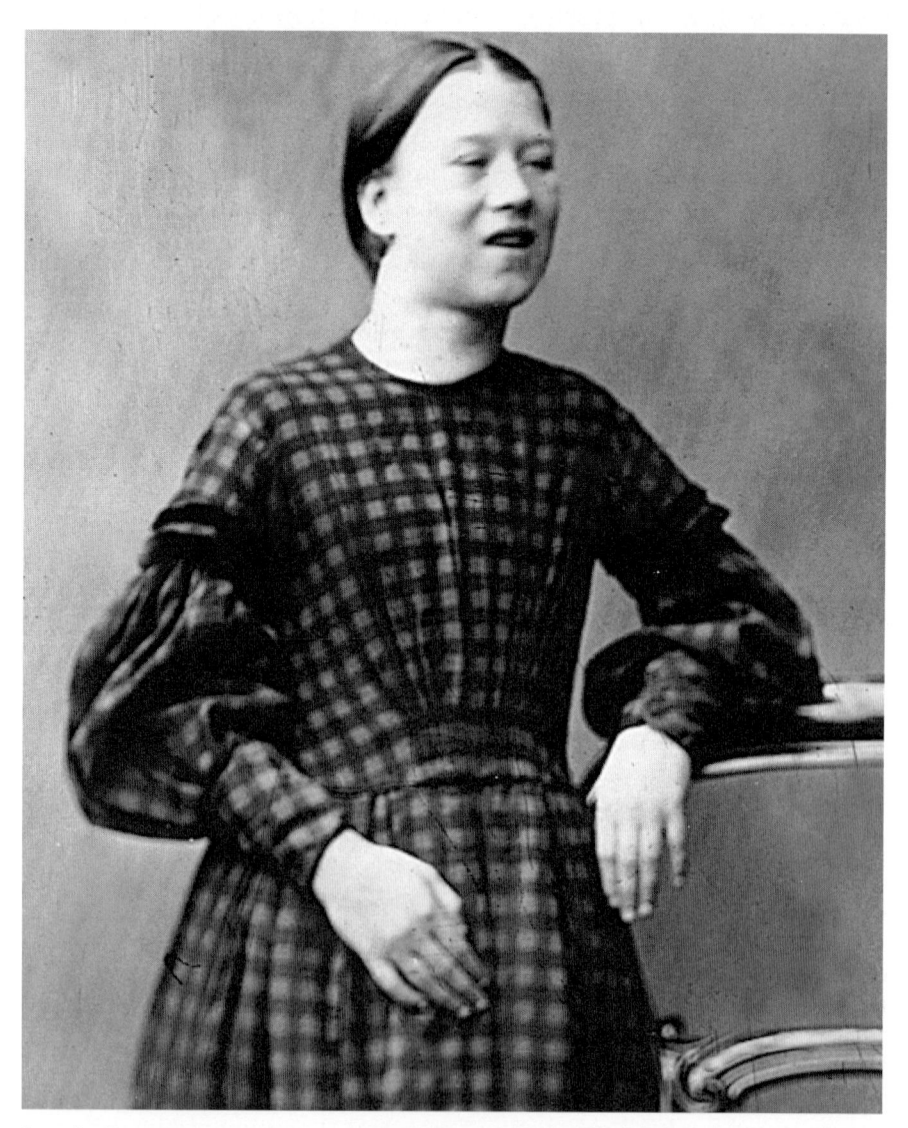

Langdon Down began to take clinical photographs in 1862. His first photograph of an Earlswood resident with Down's syndrome was this unnamed girl in the 1865 series. She was probably the first ever Down's syndrome patient to be photographed.

most interesting features of the collection of photographs is the apparently normal physical appearance of most of his photographic subjects; these are the members of the great Caucasian group of the learning disabled to whom he referred. The physical appearance of all his photographic subjects also confirms their general wellbeing. The residents of Earlswood were well-dressed, well-fed and well-cared for and the photographs support the very high standards maintained in the institution.

The 1865 series of photographs fortuitously includes a number of negatives of great interest, including photographs of his wife Mary and of Everleigh and Lilian, the Langdon Down's first two children. There is also a photograph of a brain specimen removed at autopsy during that period. No details were etched on the negative of the brain by Langdon Down and so it is unclear which of the patients who died in 1865 proved to be so important that the brain appearances were photographed and kept.

Professor Esiri has since studied the photograph and observed that the critical area of the temporal lobe is out of focus, but there is a posterior cut-off which could be suggestive of Down's syndrome[2]. There is a suggestively sharp slope to the back of the brain and the superior temporal gyrus is ill-defined. Langdon Down, in his publications on brain abnormalities, does not refer to any photographic material. When medical visitors visited Earlswood he brought them to see the individual patients and, when he made his clinical presentations at meetings, he probably passed around the developed and mounted prints rather than using the magic lantern for the projection of slide material. He probably also passed around for inspection the skull vaults which he had retained from autopsy examinations.

As a matter of interest none of his surviving 1862 negatives identifies any resident with typical signs of Down's syndrome. Perhaps M (No. 90) attracted his attention with the rather fanciful description of the Ethiopian characteristics. He described these as prominent eyes, puffy lips, retreating chin and woolly hair. N (No. 101) may have given a rather fanciful notion of the Malayan variety which he describes as having black curly hair, prominent upper jaws and capacious mouths. It was not until the 1865 series that any resident emerges with features which could fancifully be described as Aztec in appearance. The shortened forehead, prominent cheeks, deep set eyes and slightly apish nose can rather fancifully reflect this description in the photographs of an unnamed patient photographed in 1865. This, presumably was one of the early photographs of that year, the negative being in one of the Normansfield boxes beginning with negative number 6. There is no way, however, that this resident can be identified.

In the 1865 series patient number 138 and patient number 155 might be perceived as showing slightly Negroid features. An unnamed boy (190) might be regarded as having some Aztec features. The entire concept of ethnic classification however, was one which appealed to Langdon Down as being a very good idea at the time, but one which he subsequently abandoned. All that has survived of his observations in real terms was his identification of the large and relatively specific group whom he described as Mongolian, later to be designated as having Down's syndrome.

The Down's syndrome residents' Earlswood records differ from those of other residents only in so far as their faces are described as being oval. In each case they are also referred to as being affectionate and fond of music. Their external skull measurements are included without comment and the foreshortening of the head – which is shown by these measurements – is not specifically referred to in the notes, although Langdon Down referred to it in his Lettsomian Lectures.

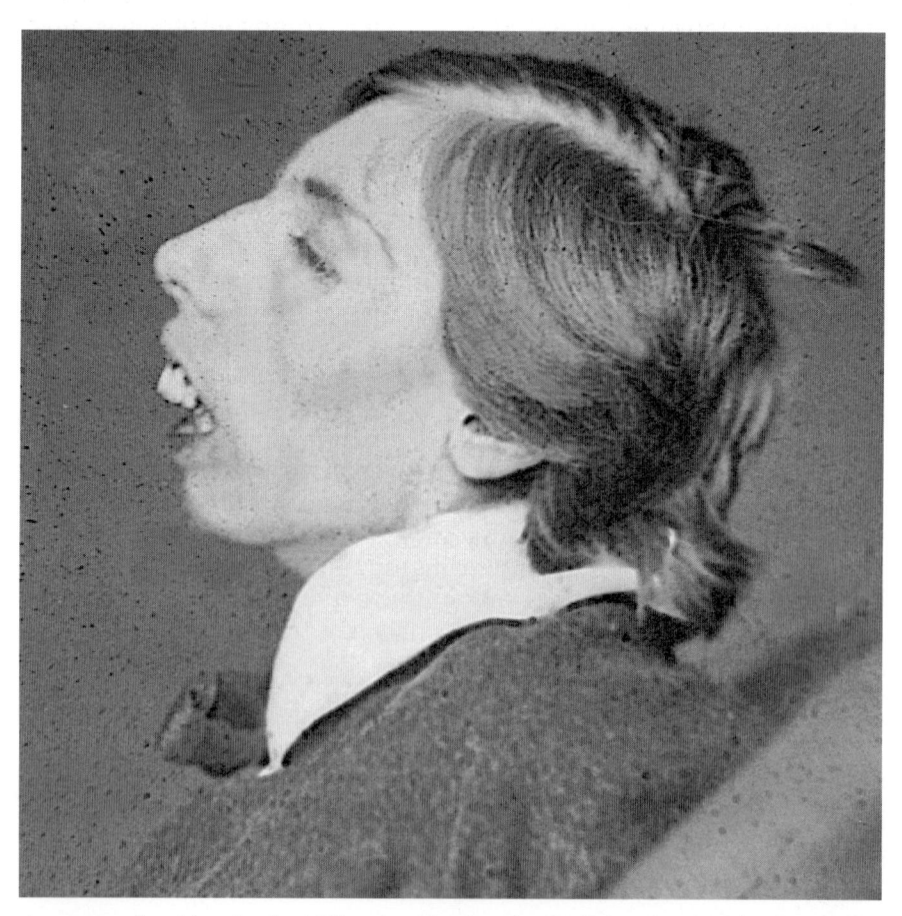

An unnamed resident in the 1865 series, showing the small foreshortened head and what Langdon Down describes as a 'slightly apish nose', with deep-set eyes, possibly his Aztec prototype.

The failure of Langdon Down to complete the photographic survey and incorporate the photographic prints in the casenotes was, no doubt, related to the enormous time content involved. If a patient moved or was uncooperative the whole process had to be started again. 'Posing chairs' existed as a means of restraining sitters for the long exposure times that were required but there is no evidence in any of Langdon Down's photographs that he used these.

The photographs incorporated in the casebooks were the second series of prints, an initial series on thin paper being unsatisfactory for gluing to the pages concerned. Casebooks for boys and girls were separate and, although there were fewer girls than boys in Earlswood (or perhaps because of this), the attachment of photographs to the clinical records is more complete in 1865 for girls than it is for boys. Langdon Down had probably not completed the pasting in when he left Earlswood in 1868. It would appear that the plan had been to clear the backlog of girls in the first instance and then to move on to the boys and men. In any event, it is most interesting to have the opportunity of actually noting the spectrum of clinical appearances of such a large number of residents and to speculate on how long it took Langdon Down to specifically identify the group which he described as 'Mongolian'.

When John Langdon Down published his 'Ethnic Classification'[2] there was no process for the printing of photographs in medical journals. The technology for the reproduction of photographs did not emerge until 1895 but photographs were, however, passed around at medical meetings. The first clinical photographs of children with learning difficulties were not published until 1895[3]. The first published photograph of a pateint with Down's syndrome was published in 1898[4]. Langdon Down could not publish his photographs in the years in which he took them and the best he could do may have been to bring his developed prints to medical meetings. The existence of his photographs almost passed unnoticed. His Earlswood negatives have been lodged in the Surrey Record Office and his Normansfield collection in the London Metropolitan Records Office, together with Reginald's 1912 series.

References

1 Esiri M. Personal Communication to author, 1997.
2 Down JL. Observations on an Ethnic Classification of Idiots. *London Hospital Reports*. 1862; **3**: 259–62.
3 Telford Smith T. Cases of spontaneous cretinism treated by thyroid extract. *J Ment Sc* 1895; **33**: 280–1.
4 Ireland WW. *Children, Idiocy and Insanity*. London: Churchill 1898.

Chapter 20

The End of a Partnership

In the winter of 1889 John Langdon Down contracted a severe bout of influenza. He was confined to bed for three months and clearly suffered from a serious and prolonged illness. He was treated with quinine, usually prescribed to reduce high temperatures and bromide, because he could not sleep, possibly due to a troublesome cough. In February of 1890 he began to take digitalis, possibly indicating that he had developed cardiac complications. He made a slow recovery and, following the illness, he was noticed to have aged considerably. He continued with his work in the London Hospital and was now an Alderman of Middlesex.

John Langdon Down was beginning to pay the price of his heavy professional and public duties and was losing momentum. The end came suddenly, but not before he had seen his sons qualified in medicine and both comfortably in line to take up his medical inheritance; before he died, Reginald and Percival were registered officially on the Normansfield licence. The new clock tower was completed in 1892 and the impressive conservatory, which still stands, was also finished in that year. He also lived to see Reginald married in 1895 and he met Percival's future fiancée. In the same year, possibly due to a premonition that all was not well, he opened a joint bank account with his wife Mary.

On Wednesday 7th October, 1896 he rose early and went to take his breakfast in Normansfield before setting out for Harley Street. He collapsed and died suddenly. His son Reginald attended him and Dr Gunther was called. Dr Gunther was later to sign the death certificate giving 'a sudden heart attack' as the cause of death. He never regained consciousness. He had been under medical supervision and, when the coroner was contacted he indicated that no inquest would be required. Langdon Down's death cast a shadow not only over Normansfield but over Hampton Wick and Kingston as well. He was a well-known local figure and the public perception was of a benevolent man who was kindly, courteous and considerate. He had made his way from humble beginnings and was respected for his perseverance[1].

When his funeral procession passed through Kingston to St Thomas's Church in Portland Square the pavements were lined with people standing in silent respect. Shops were closed and blinds drawn. So many floral tributes had been received that a separate landau was needed to convey them. Mary Langdon Down travelled in the first mourning carriage, with her son Percival and Fanny Rains, the niece who had come to be a daughter figure. When the cortège reached 81 Harley Street the procession paused and, when it finally reached the church, members of Langdon Down's staff carried the casket from the entrance to the top of the aisle. The funeral was an Anglican one. The Langdon Downs were of Nonconformist stock but changed their affiliation in 1883, the year of Everleigh's death. From then on the Normansfield chaplains were Church of England.

Mary Langdon Down could not face the public ceremony. Her distress was overwhelming and she sat in the vestry alone with her sister-in-law, devastated by the intensity of her grieving. The service was conducted by the Reverend Thompson and the text taken from the Old Testament; 'A man greatly beloved'. (Daniel 12). In his homily the Reverend spoke of John Langdon Down's Christian life and good works. Having the first part of the funeral service in St Thomas's Church gave an opportunity to the Langdon Downs' many London friends and representatives of the professional associations and hospitals to pay their respects. The Langdon Downs had taken their places in the pews at St Thomas's whenever they had spent Sundays in Harley Street, as they sometimes did. Colleagues from the London Hospital included Dr Stephen MacKenzie and Dr Hughlings Jackson and also a large number of nurses. Representatives of the British Medical Association, Hampton Wick District Council and other bodies were also present.

Langdon Down had directed that he was to be cremated and, after the homily, the casket was brought to Waterloo Station and transferred by train to Woking Crematorium. Only 10 close family members attended the cremation service, followed by a long journey from Woking to Normansfield. It was dark when the funeral party reached Normansfield, where the theatre had been set out for Langdon Down's final funeral service the following morning, which replaced the usual service of morning prayer. The urn with Langdon Down's ashes was placed on a raised platform. Above it was his picture and on a velvet cushion were laid out his hospital medals. Five obituary notices were published[2-6]. The *BMJ* wrote that Langdon Down, in living up to the highest principles himself, had gained influence over both young and old and was a powerful good[3]. The *Lancet* describes him as having spoken with the deepest feeling and with much beauty of expression on the more spiritual side of man's life [3].

Mary Langdon Down had no opportunity to heal her private wounds in peace, as Normansfield still had to be administered and the daily routine planned. The loss of her husband had affected all the staff and she had to give a lead in recalling them all to their duty of care for the residents. She ran Normansfield without her husband's advice but aided by her two sons, Reginald and

The End of a Partnership

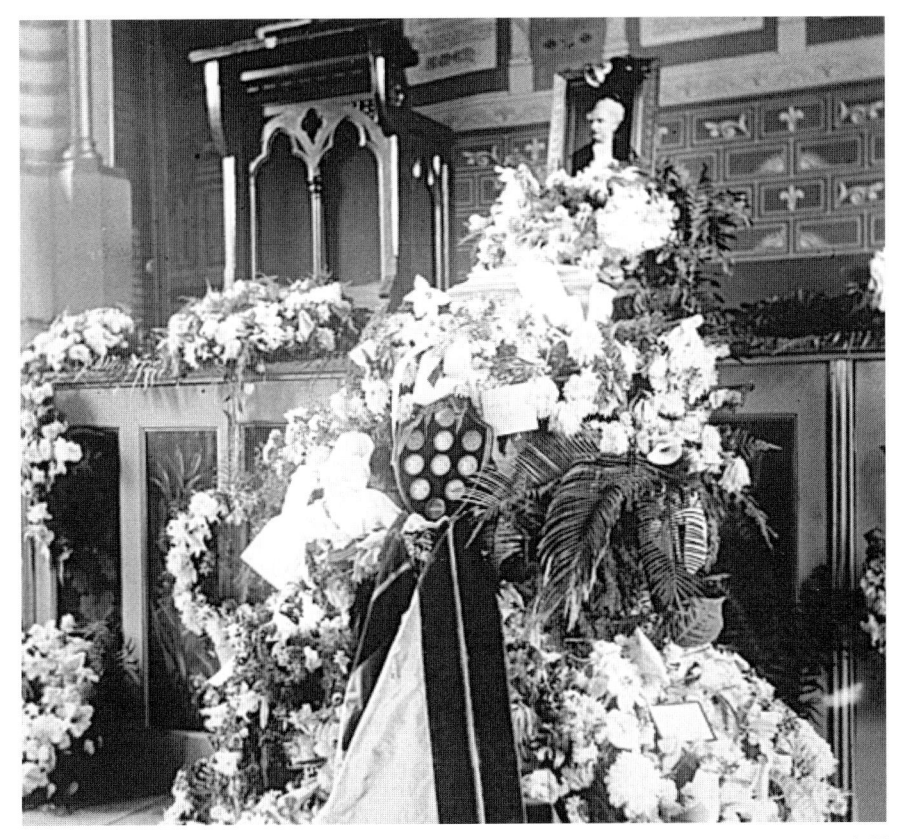

The urn containing the ashes of John Langdon Down at the funeral service in the Normansfield theatre; his hospital gold medals are on a velvet cushion. Mary died five years later and their combined ashes were scattered in Normansfield.

Percival, who were now qualified in medicine, although as yet inexperienced.

In 1899 Percival married, a happy event, but illness struck soon after when Mary developed a severe attack of influenza. There was a worse epidemic in 1900 and 10 of the residents died. 'Little Mother' continued working but she too contracted the new virulent infection. On this occasion it ran a fulminant course and she died on 5 October, 1900 of influenza and pneumonia[7]. She was cremated in Woking and her urn was also brought to Normansfield. Here it was set on a lace table-cover in the Normansfield theatre beside that of the urn containing the ashes of her husband. The front of the platform was occupied by a magnificent array of flowers and wreaths.

The funeral service was attended by over 300 people, including family, relatives, friends, doctors and their wives, members of staff and some parents. The funeral service was conducted by the hospital chaplain and the Reverend Percy Thompson, who had conducted her husband's service. He spoke of the strength and vigour of Mary's nature and character, her keen judgement, active but careful mind and tender woman's heart. Life, he said, was only a part of the human expectation. There was a life to follow where what had faithfully begun should be completed, not undone. She had begun a great work and this would continue. Although a soldier might die at his post the army would march on. They should pray that God would grant his blessing on the work that had been begun and carried on there, that it might be continued and become an even greater blessing to those who might enter its walls in the years to come. It was Mary's expressed wish that her ashes should be put with her husbands, consigned to that place which was consecrated to them, Normansfield. No stone marks the place where the couple's ashes came to be scattered. It is tempting to think that they may have been laid to rest under the mulberry tree where they often sat in their moments of relaxation.

The Langdon Downs had accumulated great wealth. On the day on which they were married, on 10 October 1860, John Langdon Down had written a simple will bequeathing all his assets to his wife Mary. A formal will, executed in August 1887, confirmed this. Mary Langdon Down managed her affairs with prudence and when she died, four years after her husband, the total estate was valued at £48,656, between £2.5 and £3 million in present day terms. The estate was to be divided equally between her sons Reginald and Percival. Their financial future was clearly assured. In comparative terms the Langdon Down estate was valued at more than twice that of Victorian Presidents and Censors of the Royal College of Physicians, whose average estates were listed as £17,500 approximately[8].

Normansfield remained under the supervision of the Langdon Down family. Reginald's and Percival's wives both took over where Mary Langdon Down had left off. Reginald lived to the grand age of 89; after his death his daughter Stella, later Lady Brain, continued working at Normansfield. Percival was only 58 when he died but his medically qualified daughter, Molly, and his son Norman played their part, along with Lady Brain, in continuing the Normansfield tradition. Norman was the last of the Langdon Down Medical Superintendents; he retired in 1970.

References

1   *Surrey Comet*. 10 October and 17 October, 1896.
2   Obituary. *BMJ* 1896; **2**: 1170–1.
3   Obituary. *Lancet* 1896; **2**: 1104–5.
4   Obituary. *J Ment Sc* 1897; **43**: 213.
5   Obituary. *Lond Hosp Gaz* 1896; **1**: 64–6.
6   Obituary. *Pharm J* 1896; **57**: 326–30.
7   *Surrey Comet*. 6 October, 1901.
8   Peterson MD. *The Medical Profession in Mid-Victorian London*. California: University of California Press, 1978.

Chapter 21

Fame after Death

Over the years after Langdon Down's original description of 'Mongolism' as a specific type of learning disability and the adoption of the term as the appropriate designation, the importance of the original classification gradually became recognized. When Bertram Hill wrote of 'Mongolism and its pathology'[1] in 1908 he referred to Langdon Down's description and mentioned him by name, also indicating at the same time that Down's ethnic classification of mental enfeeblement had by then been abandoned. As Down himself had abandoned it, Bertram Hill was simply recognizing the importance of the description as an empirical observation.

George Shuttleworth in an address to medical students in Manchester entitled 'Clinical lecture on idiocy and imbecility[2]' wrote of the 'Mongol' or 'Kalmuc' type who constituted 3% of his cases. He also referred to Langdon Down's Ethnic Classification and listed the Mongolian type as being 'scrofulous'; the use of the word suggests an association with tuberculosis. He regarded Mongolian children as being, to an extent, unfinished in foetal development. Shuttleworth went on to repeat what Langdon Down had already observed – that the affected group of children were very susceptible to cold, had very good imitative powers, were often very fond of music and could dance and drill well but that, as a rule, died of tuberculosis before reaching the age of 20.

Gradually, Down was being given more and more credit for the importance of what he had noted. Sometimes this was done without attribution as, for instance, in Tredgold's paper on amentia in the *Practitioner* in 1908[3] and at a later stage in Penrose's paper in the *British Medical Bulletin* in 1961 which was simply entitled 'Mongolism'[4]. Dr Rainsford also used Downs' definition in his paper 'Twenty years experience of imbeciles of the Mongolian type' published in the *Journal of Medical Science* in 1917[5].

The final official accolade of international recognition came in 1961. The importance of Langdon Down's role was recognized in a prestigious letter to the *Lancet*. The letter was signed by 20 international experts, including some of the most famous workers in the field of disability. The letter read:

Sir,

It has long been recognized that the terms 'Mongolian Idiocy', 'Mongolism', 'Mongoloid' etc. as applied to a specific type of mental deficiency have misleading connotations. The occurrence of this anomaly among Europeans and their descendants is not related to the segregation of genes derived from Asians; it's appearance among members of Asian populations suggests such ambiguous designations as 'Mongol Mongoloid'; the increasing participation of Chinese and Japanese investigators in the study of the condition imposes on them the use of an embarrassing term. We urge, therefore, that the expressions which imply a racial aspect of the condition be no longer used.

Some of the undersigned are inclined to replace the term Mongolism by such designations as 'Langdon Down anomaly', or 'Down's syndrome or anomaly', or 'congenital acromicria'. Several others believe that this is an appropriate time to introduce the term 'trisomy 21 anomaly', which would include cases of simple trisomy as well as translocations. It is hoped that agreement on a specific phrase will soon crystallize once the term 'Mongolism' has been abandoned[6].

Gordon Allen and Professor Penrose masterminded the letter and organized signatories from both the UK and US[7]. Those involved were all experts in the field of disability and, in particular, Down's syndrome. They included Bender, author of a book on Mongolism and cretinism and part of a group studying the chromosomal abnormality involved; Ford, one of the original laboratory workers who had developed the techniques for the recognition of chromosomes; Lejeune and Turpin who, together, had first stated with certainty that the extra chromosome 21 was characteristic of the condition; and Warkany, the author of a textbook on congenital malformations and the world expert on syndromes and maldevelopment.

Penrose himself had extended the observations on the palmar creases first made by Reginald Langdon Down and went on to review the pattern of ridge formation in the skin of the hands and feet. He identified the importance of maternal age and went on to describe the manner in which Down's syndrome could result from the entrapment of a portion of a chromosome on to a normal pair. This could also produce a clinical picture of Trisomy 21, although the total chromosome count was normal. Penrose and Allen had agreed between them that the term Mongolism should be replaced and organized the process which was to follow. Another of the signatories was Norman Langdon Down, the third generation of medical Langdon Downs to be involved in the family institution at Normansfield. Penrose contacted him to ask if the family would agree to the proposal to link the family name with the syndrome and he agreed. On the published letter his initial is actually misprinted as 'W', but it is to Norman that it refers.

The editor of the *Lancet* accepted the new designation. He said that the term derived from Langdon Down's observations on an ethnic description of idiots, in which he wrote that the great Mongolian family had many representatives. The editor accepted that Down had given a good description of the appearance of these patients in later childhood. For these reasons he ruled that 'Down's syndrome is an appropriate alternative for Mongolian Idiocy until the chromosome abnormalities in the disorder have been fully elucidated and a new scientific descriptive term could be coined'[8].

The new designation was accepted without dispute, unsurprisingly given the very prestigious support which had been accorded to the renaming of the condition. The decision was probably taken by Dr Ian Munro, deputy editor, who then had editorial responsibility for the correspondence section and ultimately went on to become editor of the *Lancet*. His decision to designate the condition as an eponymous one attracted some private criticism, but he never revised his position[9].

There were only two rather lightweight objections registered, from Dr Spalding of the Churchill Hospital in Oxford and from Dr Papworth of London. They were in favour of retaining the established designation of Mongolian idiocy, but the ruling of the editor was accepted de facto and, although the underlying chromosome abnormality and its variations came to be fully defined, the term Down's syndrome was thereafter commonly used rather than trisomy 21. The logic of this convention is that, while most patients with the condition do indeed have an extra chromosome 21, there are some other variants of this particular chromosome which may also produce the clinical picture and so the use of a broader descriptive term remains justified.

The designation was confirmed by the World Health Organization in 1965. The representative of the People's Republic of Mongolia approached the Director-General and said that they objected to the use of the descriptive 'Mongolian Idiot' as it was derogatory to them. Partly as a result of this Down's syndrome was adopted as the official definition[10], and remains so today. There was an international symposium on 'Mongolism' in 1967. This was chaired by Lord Russell Brain, who gave an introductory account of the contribution of Langdon Down to the subject. Lord Brain had married Stella Langdon Down, Reginald's daughter. He was naturally very proud of the family name and accomplishments and gave a detailed account of Langdon Down's work in the field. He referred to the condition as 'Down's syndrome' and his undoubted support for the eponymous designation again set the seal of authority on the use of the new descriptive term. There is, as yet, no consensus on the choice between 'Down's syndrome' as originally suggested and 'Down syndrome' as the preferred usage. The former is widely used in the United Kingdom and the latter in the US.

In spite of the worldwide acceptance of his status Langdon Down is almost a forgotten man. There are few permanent memorials in his honour, apart from the plaque on the facade of Normansfield, the street names in Torpoint and Teddington and the commemorative bust in Richmond Council offices (for the services for people with learning difficulties). His only biography until now has been in German[12] and only a handful of tributes have been paid to him in the medical and social work literature[13-20]. A man who contributed so much deserves more recognition from the world at large.

References

1. Bertram Hill. Mongolism and its pathology. *W Quart J Med* 1908; **2**: 49–68.
2. Shuttleworth G. Clinical lecture on idiocy and imbecility. *BMJ* 1886; **1**: 183–6.
3. Tredgold AF. Amentia. *Practitioner* 1903; **2**: 354–82.
4. Penrose LS. Mongolism. *Brit Med Bull* 1961; **17**: 184–9.
5. Rainsford A. A Review of the Admissions of Imbeciles of the Mongolian Type During the Last Twenty Years. *J Ment Sc* 1917; **44**: 238–41.
6. Allen G, Benda CJ, *et al*. Letters. *Lancet* 1961; **1**: 775.
7. Polani P. Personal Communication to author, 1996.
8. Editorial Comment. *Lancet* 1961; **2**: 935.
9. Munro I. Personal Communication to author, 1964.
10. Howard-Jones N. On the diagnostic term 'Down's syndrome'. *Medical History* 1979; **22**: 102–4.
11. Brain Lord R. Historical Introduction. In: Wolstenholme GEW, Porter R. *Mongolism*. Ciba Foundation Study Group No 25, 1967: 1–5.
12. Pies N. *John Langdon Hayden Langdon-Down (1826–1896). Ein pionier der Sozialpadiatrie*. Karlsruhe: G Braun, 1996.
13. Sakula A. Royal Earlswood hospital: a historical sketch. *J Roy S Med* 1998; **81**: 107–8.
14. Dunn P. Dr Langdon Down (1828–1896) and 'mongolism'. *Arch Dis Child* 1991; **66**: 827–8.
15. Sullivan T. John Langdon Down. In: *the Founders of Child Neurology*. San Francisco: Norman Publishers, 1990.
16. Beighton P, Beighton G. Down Syndrome. In: *The Man Behind the Syndrome*. London: Springer Verlag, 1986.
17. Birch A. Down's Syndrome. John Langdon Haydon Langdon-Down 1828–1896. *Practitioner* 1973; **210**: 171–2.
18. Brown GH. *Lives of the Fellows of the Royal College of Physicians of London 1826–1925*. London: Royal College of Physicians, 1955.
19. Tollis D. Who was ... Down? *Nursing Times* 1995; **91**: 6 1.
20. Zihni L. *The History of the Relation Between the Concept and Treatment of People with Down's syndrome in Britain and America from 1866–1967*. Unpublished D. Phil. thesis. University of London, 1990.

―――――――――――― Appendix 1 ――――――――――――

The indenture of John Langdon Down to his father as an apothecary. The original has no punctuation marks. (Courtesy of Dr Michael Brain).

The Indenture Witnesseth That

John Langdon Haydon Down doth put himself apprentice to Joseph Almond Down apothecary of Torpoint Cornwall to learn his Art and with him after the Manner of an Apprentice to serve from the first day of January eighteen hundred and forty nine unto the full end and term of five years from thence next following to be fully complete and ended during which Term the said apprentice his Master faithfully shall serve his secrets keep his lawful commands every where gladly he shall do no damage to his said master nor see to be done of others but to his Power shall tell or forthwith give warning to his said master of the same he shall not ways the goods of his said master nor lend them unlawfully to any he shall not commit fornication nor contract Matrimony within the said term shall not the Cards or Dice Tables or any other unlawful games whereby his said master may have any loss with his own goods or others during the said Term without License of his said master he shall neither buy nor sell he shall not haunt Taverns or Playhouses nor absent himself from his said master s service day or night unlawfully. But all things as a faithful Apprentice he shall behave himself towards his said master and all during his said Term and the said Joseph Almond Down in consideration of the services of the said John Langdon Haydon Down doth hereby contract and agree to instruct his said apprentice sufficient Meat Drink Lodging and all other Necessaries during the said Term.

And for the true performance of all and every the said Covenants and the Agreements either of the said Parties bindeth himself unto the other by these Presents in Witness whereof the said Parties bindeth himself unto the other by those Presents in Witness whereof the Parties above named to these Indentures interchangeably have put their Hands and Seals the first day of January and in the twelfth year of the reign of our Sovereign Lady Victoria by the Grace of God of the United Kingdom of Great Britain and Ireland Queen Defender of the Faith and in the year of our Lord One Thousand Eight Hundred and Forty Nine.

J A Down   J L H Down

N.B. The Indenture Covenant Article or Contract must bear date the day it is executed and what Money or other thing is given or contacted from with the Clerk or Apprentice must be inserted in Words at Length otherwise the Indenture will be void the Master or Mistress forfeit Fifty Pounds and another Penalty and the Apprentice be disabled to follow the trade or be made Free.

Witnesses

John B Rogers   P W Puck

---Appendix 2---

The Normansfield Theatre
John Earl

The addition of an Entertainment Hall to Normansfield in 1879 was not, in itself, an exceptional event. Any large Victorian residential institution would have been likely to have a multi-purpose assembly and meeting place which could serve the community as a ballroom, concert room or occasional theatre and, if no purpose-built chapel existed, also as a place of worship. Asylums, in particular, where the staff worked for long periods in an enclosed environment, had a pressing need for in-house entertainment.

Most surviving recreation halls in asylums tend to be useful rather than beautiful. A few – for example, those at Stanley Royd Hospital in Wakefield, St Nicholas Hospital, Gosforth, near Newcastle upon Tyne and Claybury Hospital, Woodford Bridge – are of more than ordinary ambition, but Normansfield stands head and shoulders above them all.

Normansfield's Entertainment Hall is, in fact, one of the most remarkable private theatres in Britain[1]. Reports of its opening describe it as having 'all the appliances of a well-equipped theatre, with green room, dressing rooms and scenic arrangements... capital stage, footlights, drop scene...everything complete'[1]. The Commissioners in Lunacy observing, in 1882, on the excellent accommodation at Normansfield, added that it had 'a fine theatre for dramatic performances, concerts and dances'[1]. There was also a spacious Kindersaal in the room under the auditorium, which served as a wet weather playroom and skating rink[2].

The normal miscellany of uses had to be accommodated in the hall but, whilst in most asylums theatrical activity was, at best, occasional, at Normansfield it was intensive. The importance John Langdon Down attached to children's games, entertainment and drama as a means to stimulating intelligence is dealt with in Chapter 12. In this respect, a theatre was essential to his Normansfield regime. Lady Brain recalled how 'there was every chance for any patient (or staff) who so wished and was able, to sing, dance, recite or act in unison or solo. Every Thursday from 6 to 7 pm 'The Entertainment' took place in the hall where everyone met for their hour's enjoyment. Programmes were printed each week on the Normansfield Press... and it was a great pride to be on the bill'.

What might loosely be called therapeutic uses of the stage could, however, have been accommodated in a more modestly equipped room, but the Langdon Down family were keen on the drama for its own sake. They could afford the very best standard of provision in their own theatre which was (apart from its necessarily flat auditorium floor) in many ways a miniature version of a professional theatre. It was always in regular use for the Langdon Downs' own amateur productions and rehearsals, mostly farces, comedies and burlesques and, in 1891, the family and a few of their friends formed the Genesta Amateur Dramatic Club, with Mrs Langdon Down as 'acting manager'. The club grew rapidly in numbers and popularity and, for 19 years, presented four or five productions a year – plays, pantomimes, concerts and the occasional Gilbert and Sullivan Opera – until, in 1910, they moved their activities to Surbiton.

The theatre was designed by the architect of all the early additions to the original house, Rowland Plumbe. It appears to be the only theatre he was ever called upon to design and, in most respects, his achievement is impressive. The hall itself, with its open-trussed roof and decorative central gas sunburner (a device which provided both light and extract ventilation) is well-constructed; the proscenium, however, is nothing short of spectacular. It is an elaborate polychromatic composition of great splendour and equal to the best private and public decorative work of the 1870s and 80s.

The stage is provided with a groove system, a method of scene changing which was common to all English theatres from the seventeenth to the late nineteenth century, but now survives in working order in only two places, Wakefield and Normansfield. This allowed scene changes and transformations to be made rapidly, in full view of the audience, by sliding wing flats on from the side, while simultaneously changing the painted back scene. The Normansfield stage not only still operates on this system, but also has an extraordinary collection of scenery made specially for it. This collection of around 100 pieces of high quality painted stock scenery is unique in Britain.

The Theatre is included in the statutory list of buildings of special architectural or historic interest at an unusually high grade (II*) reflecting its outstanding national importance. The scenery, sadly, cannot itself be protected by listing, but the interest of the building would be seriously damaged if it were to be lost or removed.

The sale of Normansfield by the Health Authority has focused minds on the need for a solution to the problem of preserving Langdon Down's remarkable theatre. A way must be found to keep the building and its contents in an appropriate use under curatorial care. Its presentation to the public will need to reveal and explain its architectural, theatrical and archaeological importance. Most importantly, Dr Langdon Down and his work with the learning disabled should be celebrated here.

John Earl
August 1998

Reference

1 Earl J. *Dr John Langdon-Down and the Normansfield Theatre.* Twickenham: Borough of Twickenham Local History Society, 1997.
2 Commissioners in Lunacy Report, 1882.

Index

Abbreviations:
JLD   John Langdon Down
RLD   Reginald Langdon Down

Abbiss, Mr   55, 62
Allen, Gordon   200
Anderson, Elizabeth Garrett   163
Andrew, Thomas   88
Apothecaries Act (1815)   10, 23
Apothecaries, Worshipful Society   9–10, 21–2, 23
Ashby, Lord   30
Athenaeum Club   121

Banting, William   69
Bell, Jacob   19
Bicêtre Hospital (Paris)   34
Bigwood, James   141
Bigwood, Mouche   141
Blumenbach, Friedrich   183
BMJ (British Medical Journal)   88
Bradley, James   124, 125
Brady, Cheyne   52
Brain, Lady Stella   141, 142, 198, 205
Brain, Lord Christopher   188
Brain, Lord Russell   141, 147, 201
Briggs, Caroline & William   140
Broadbent, Henry   42
Brock company   140
Broderers' Company   121
Brush, Edward   136
Bucknill, JC   176
Buxton, Charles   45

Caldecott, Dr   170
Carroll, Sir George   30
Champneys, Reverend Canon   39
Channing, Walter   161
Christian Union article   100–3
Clark, Andrew   62–3
Clark, James   38, 73, 180–1
Cleveland, Jane Jarvey   141
Colchester Asylum   88
Coleman, Dr   92
Coleman, Matthew   7, 8
Cone, Tom   136

Conolly, John   34, 36, 37, 38
  beliefs   32–3, 179–83
  death   67
  influence on JLD   43, 49, 180–3
  interest in ethnology   129, 182
  meets Séguin   34, 180
Cooper, John   63
Cornelia de Lange syndrome   130, 165
Coutts, Baroness   111
Crayon, Christopher   31
Crellin, Mary *see* Down, Mary
Crellin, Philip (junior)   4, 15, 19, 20, 23, 42, 140
Crellin, Philip (senior)   42, 43
Crellin, Sarah   20, 26, 41, 43–4, 140, 188
Crookshank, FG   132

Darenth Asylum   143
Darenth Training Schools   88
Darwin, Charles   175
Davies, Herbert   21, 131, 159
Diamond, Hugh Welch   182
Dictionary of Medicine (Quain, 1882)   53, 133
Diplock, Dr   125
Diseases of Children (Goodhart, 1888)   136
Disraeli, Benjamin   176
Down & Son   1, 3–4, 7, 9
Down Brothers   9, 12
Down, Everleigh (son)   79, 116
  birth   56
  childhood/youth   123, 139–40
  death/burial   58–9, 123–7, 184
  photographed by JLD   188, 191
Down, Hannah (mother)   2, 5, 20
Down, Henry (brother)   12
Down, Henry (nephew)   12
Down, John Langdon
  birth   1
  childhood/early life   1–5

Down, John Langdon (*continued*)
  death/funeral   97, 195–8
  Earlswood appointment   41–74, 180–2
  Ethnic Classification   130–2, 158, 178–9, 182, 189–93
  illnesses   15, 96–7, 195
  Lettsomian lectures   6, 47, 129, 134, 135, 157–73
  London Hospital Address (1864)   88–92
  London Hospital appointments   24–7, 61–4, 66, 83, 92
  marriage   42
  medical studies   19–27
  membership of societies   184
  missing records mystery   71–3
  name change   77–8
  Normansfield era   77–84, 115–21
  pharmaceutical training   7–8, 10–12, 203–4
  photographs of   187–93
  prize essay   15–17, 27
  publications   98, 129–32, 157
  Social Science Congress lecture (1867)   83–8, 98
  temperament   44
  trips abroad   123, 140–1
  views on
    alcohol   2, 48, 54
    Darwinism   175–7
    Down's syndrome   131–2, 149–50, 158–9
    medical ethics   89–91
    people with disability   17, 25, 85–9, 97–9, 157–73
    phrenology   132–3, 159–60, 170
  will   198
Down, Joseph Almond (father)   1–2, 4, 5, 22, 23
Down, Joseph Kelland (grandfather)   4–5
Down, Kelland (brother)   2, 9
Down, Lilian (daughter)   56–60, 191
Down, Mary (wife)   41–2, 55, 92
  children   55–60, 74, 78
  Christian Union editorial   103
  courtship   26–7
  death/funeral   107, 197–8
  Earlswood work   43, 69–71
  Normansfield work   82, 83, 98, 107–14, 116–21
  personality   107, 113–14
  poetry   59–60, 113
  will   98
Down, Richard (brother)   1, 2, 3, 4, 5, 7, 9, 12
Down, Sarah *see* Crellin, Sarah
Down Street (Teddington)   1
Down's syndrome   47, 87, 129–37
  designation   199–202
  individual cases   82, 101, 150–6
  JLD on   131–2, 149–50, 158–9
  JLD's photographs   189–93
  RLD on   132, 143–5, 179
Duchenne, Dr C   166
Duncan, PM   134
Dunn, Robert   178–9
Durant, Susan   4

Earlswood Asylum   27, 29–40, 83
  early problems   34–8
  JLD's tenure   41–74, 180–2
  museum   129, 169
Education and Training for the Feeble in Mind (Down, 1876)   83–8, 98
Ellis, Lady   92
Encyclopedia of the Diseases of Children (1891)   136
epidemics   64–6, 95–6, 153
epilepsy   84, 164–5
Esiri, M   191
Ethnic Classification   130–2, 158, 178–9, 182
  photographic studies   189–93
ethnology   129, 182–3
  see also phrenology
Everett, Frederick   71
Everett, Mrs   70

Fagg, Miss M   51, 69–70
Faraday, Michael   13
Farmer, Dr   125
Farr White, Mr   125
Fell, Dr   143
Forbes, Sir John   29, 33–4, 36, 37, 38
Ford, Jane (sister)   42, 178
Ford, Reverend David   42, 178
Fownes, George   9
Fraser, Robert   135

galvanism 166–7
Gee, Samuel 111
Genesta Amateur Dramatic Club 117, 120, 206
Giessen University (Germany) 19
Gilpin, Charles 30
Goodhart, JF 136
Grabham, Dr GW 73, 130
Great Ormond Street Hospital 134, 136, 188
Griesinger, W 134
Guggenbuhl, Johann 29
Gunther, Dr T 104, 124–7, 153, 195

Harley, G 68
Harley Street practice 78
Hibbs, Mr 140
Hill, Bertram 199
Howe, Samuel 177
Hutchinson, Mr J 125

idiots savants 167–70
International Medical Congress (1881) 111

Jackson, Hughlings 39, 63, 66, 79, 196
Jacobi, Abraham 111
Jolly, Miss 29

Keeling, Mr 160
Kidd, Frederick 64
Kraft, I 180

Langdon Down, Elspie 141
Langdon Down, John *see* Down, John Langdon
Langdon Down, Mary *see* Down, Mary
Langdon Down, Molly 147, 198
Langdon Down, Norman 141, 147, 198, 200
Langdon Down, Percival (son) 79, 123, 139–48
  birth 77
  coming of age 12, 112, 140
  death 198
  marriage 141
  medical work 146–7
  sailing ventures 81–2
  theatrical interests 116–17
Langdon Down, Reginald (son) 79, 139–48
  death 198
  death of Everleigh 123–7
  death of JLD 195
  on Down's syndrome 132, 143–5, 179
  marriage 141
  medical interests 143–6
  photographic survey 146, 188
  resigns MRCP 147–8
  sailing ventures 81–2
  theatrical interests 116–17
Langdon Down, Tony 141
Lankester, Edwin 123
Lankester, Mrs Phoebe 123
Lawrence, William 22
Lee, Walter 78, 140
Lejeune, JM 200
Lettsom, John Coakley 157
Lettsomian lectures 46, 47, 129, 134, 135, 157–73
Liebig, Professor 19–20
Little, WJ 20, 33, 38, 62, 63, 67
Little's disease 33, 172
Llewellyn, David 89–90
London Hospital 20–7
  JLD's appointments 24–7, 61–4, 66, 83, 92
  London Hospital Address (1864) 89–92
London Hospital Reports 65, 130
Lunnon, Ray 188

MacKenzie, Morell 66
Mackenzie, Stephen 145, 196
Maxwell, Dr 36–7, 48, 167
Meadows, A 136
Medical Society of London 157, 184
Mental Deficiency Act (1913) 88
Middlesex County Pauper Lunatic Asylum 179
Miller, James 65
Mitchell, Arthur 134–5
Mongol in our Midst, The (Crookshank, 1924) 132
'Mongolian' Type 47, 87, 129–37, 158
  Ethnic Classification 130–2, 158, 178–9, 182

'Mongolian' Type (*continued*)
  term replaced 199–202
  see also Down's syndrome
Morel, Benedict 177
Munro, Ian 201

National Society for Women's Suffrage 163
Nelson, Sir Thomas 121, 125
Normansfield 77–84, 95–106
  Down's syndrome patients 82, 149–56
  Mary Langdon Down's role 107–14
  Normansfield Theatre 115–21, 205–7
  official enquiry (1974) 142
  photographic work 187–93
  under NHS 141, 142

Odom, Herbert 176

Papworth, Dr MH 201
Peacock, Dr 159
Penrose, LS 199–200
Pereira, Jonathon 8, 12
Pharmaceutical Society 1, 8, 9, 10, 19
photography 146, 187–93
phrenology 132–3, 159–60, 170, 182–3
Plumbe, Ebenezer 96
Plumbe, Mrs 96, 157
Plumbe, Rowland 29, 96, 206
postmortem examinations 46–7
Prader–Willi syndrome 160, 170–3
Pullen, James Henry 68, 167–70
Pullen, William Arthur 169

Quain, R 53, 133

Rains, Fanny 42, 196
Rains, John 42
Rainsford, A 199
Ramsbotham, Francis 24–5, 38, 161
Redwood, Theophilus 8, 9, 10, 14, 16, 19, 20
Reed, Andrew 29–33, 96, 180

Richards, BW 136
Ritchie, Ewing 31
Roach, Charles 125
Rothschild, Baron 30
Royal Albert Asylum (Lancaster) 145
Royal College of Surgeons 22
Royal Earlswood Asylum *see* Earlswood Asylum
Royal Earlswood Museum 129, 169
Royal Pharmaceutical Society 1, 8, 9, 10, 19
Royal Society 16
Ruddick, Miss 64–5

Sanders, Mr 190
Séguin, Edouard 34, 67–8, 134, 180, 182
Shepherd, Richard 127
Shuttleworth, George 136, 145, 199
Simmons, Ken 189
Social Science Congress (1867) 83
  JLD's lecture 83–8, 98
Spalding, Dr JMK 201
Stanley, Edward 22
Stewart Asylum (Dublin) 64, 67
Stromeyer (German surgeon) 33

Tamesis Sailing Club 81
Tanner, TH 136
Thelwall, J 176
Thompson, Anthony Todd 8
Thompson, Reverend Percy 196, 197–8
thyroid deficiency 132, 163
Ticehurst 113
Torpoint 1, 3
Tottenham, Henry 139
Travers, Benjamin 22
Tredgold, AF 136, 145, 199
trisomy-21 201
  see also Down's syndrome
Turnbull, Ruth 141
Turpin, R 200

Walker, Mrs 70
Welbeck Street practice 77–8
Wells, Spencer 111

West, Charles 134, 135–6, 162, 165, 178
Westall, Dr 71–2, 73
West's syndrome 172
Whateley, Richard 176

Wilkinson, Norman 77
Willard, AW 134
Wright, David 52, 74

Zihni, L 183